Lady
in the
Red Dress
A Personal Story of a
Woman with Heart Disease

by
Lois Trader
with Robert W. Cole

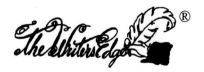

For Information:
The Writer's Edge Press and Center for Staff Development
A Division of The Writer's Edge Press
1306 Merrimont Avenue
Kings Mountain, North Carolina 28086
Telephone 704-734-0677
www.writersedgepress.com

Printed in the United States of America

Catawba Publishing Co.
5945 Orr Rd., Suite F
Charlotte, NC 28213
www.catawbapublishing.com

Trader, Lois
Lady in Red Dress: A Personal Story of a Woman with Heart Disease
Lois Trader with Robert W. Cole
ISBN: 978-0-9791767-0-8 or ISBN 0-9791767-0-0

Publisher: J. Allen Queen
Executive Editor: Robert W. Cole
Copy Editing: Sheila Way-Middleton
Typesetting and Design: Victoria Voelker
Cover Design: LouAnn Lamb
Sales and Distribution: Patsy Queen
Advertising and Marketing: Heather Thompson

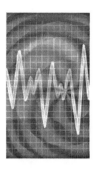

Approximately *144 million women* live in the United States.
More than *8 million* of those *144 million women* are living with heart disease.
Of that group of *8 million women*,
500,000 women will die from heart disease this year.

One woman every minute.
Take a minute to think about that.
These are harsh facts.

Cardiovascular disease is the number-one killer of women.
Then there is *me*. Lois Trader — a woman with heart disease.
And I have a story that you need to read.

Dedication

This book is dedicated to all the women who are not able to be here because heart disease didn't just interrupt their life, as it did mine. Heart disease took it.

To my father, who did not have the opportunity to live long enough to outlive heart disease. If you know in Heaven that I have inherited your genes, you also know I have always missed you and I am thankful I knew without a shadow of doubt that you loved me.

Table of Contents

Acknowledgments

To my dad, Pete Schuyler, who is mentioned in this book as my mother's husband. Pete is the dad God blessed me and with for the past 20 years. Your strength, friendship, generosity, kindness, and everlasting teaching has helped me write this book, learn to poach an egg at 50, and believe that no situation, sickness, or incident has to be the final one. I will love you for all eternity.

To my mom, Anita Schuyler. "To have and to hold, in sickness and in health" — we hear that at weddings, but I believe it should also be said at a baby's birth. As a mother, we are there for our children through it all. Whether our children understand it, have to learn it on their own, or don't communicate with us, we love them and always want the best for them. Mom, you are a wonderful example of a mother, grandmother, and great-grandmother's love. I cherish your love, example, and friendship, especially as I enter this stage of my life.

To my husband, Timothy (Hubba). Wow, haven't we been on a long ride together! I clearly remember the day I first saw you. I was 14 and you were 17. How blessed I am that the strength, looks, and biggest shoulders I'd ever seen are still as perfect to me as on that first day I saw you. Thank you for 30 years of marriage, and many years of loving you before that. From that punky freshman to the big senior on campus, you will forever be my sweetheart.

To my daughters, Bethany Ruth, Cortney Rose, and Michal Renee. At times in my life I didn't know if my heart could expand to include all the love, pleasure, and passion you have brought me. And at other times, I didn't know if my heart could heal after being broken for you. I always wanted the power to make things perfect in your lives. Now I realize that you are the beautiful individuals you are because I didn't have that power. I'm thankful, because though I never wanted you to see me sick, never wanted you to go through some of the hard times we have shared as a family, I know that you could have never become the caring, kind, lovely, loving young women you are today without it. There is nothing you will ever do that can separate our hearts. (Proverbs 4:23: "Above all else, guard your hearts, because it is the wellspring of life.") The desire to be beautiful is an ageless longing. I know that I have been a tiring example of a woman who is never satisfied to just sit and relax — always striving to do more, be more, look better, be better, but I feel so privileged to see that where I might have lacked as a mother, your own hearts filled in. You are all so very beautiful.

To Bob Cole, my co-author, and Faye Zucker, my friend. Thank you for listening to me that wonderful evening at my home, taking the time to listen to my vision and bringing this book into fruition. You have become so important to me, to my heart.

Finally, to Dr. Warren Johnston (Dave). I respect you so much. The first radio show we did together was the turning point in my goal to reach women with the message that they can, should, need to learn about their number-one killer: heart disease. I love that I did not know who you were, and yet you were so gracious and encouraging. The saying, "You've got my back" fits our relationship, but I need to tweak it a bit: "You've got my heart." Thank you for being my personal cardiologist, friend, mentor, and truly an example of a person who goes far beyond what he is expected to do. You heal other people's hearts because yours is so big.

Preface

I'm in the office, my favorite room, with dinner already prepared for my husband of 29 years. It's quiet except for the most welcomed interruptions: my oldest daughter's phone calls describing my grandchildren's most recent accomplishments, my middle daughter's emails about her baby on the way, and my youngest daughter's adventures with substitute teaching.

I feel a slight pain in my upper back — probably due to sitting too long at the computer — but it's much harder for me to dismiss such pains than it used to be. It's still difficult for me to comprehend that I have coronary artery disease, and that a stent in my left descending artery is keeping me alive.

A two-time survivor of life-threatening disease, and a woman who has lived through bankruptcy — not only financially but physically, psychologically, and spiritually — I know what it is to be bankrupt in every way. I have risen above these circumstances; my passion now is to give other women the courage to do the same.

I have been a physically fit, successful, positive, driven young woman. I have been a speaker on women's issues for the past 20 years. The willingness to show who I am has allowed me the opportunity to speak to women all over the United States, to meet with Muhammad Ali, the Prime Minister of Israel, President Reagan, and prominent ministers and civic leaders.

This book is a personal journey of being diagnosed with heart disease as a young woman — and learning to live with it. I offer practical steps to guide the reader to become healthier physically, psychologically, and spiritually. I examine the reasons why heart disease is the number-one killer of American women. Unfortunately, it is more than just a matter of plaque in our arteries.

Since 1908 the leading cause of death among American women has been heart disease. Since 1985 more women than men have died from heart disease. Two decades! Are we too busy, after fighting for justice in the workplace, to care for our hearts? Are we too exhausted to fight for our equality within the medical community? Women's lib certainly has come a long way, but since its advent we have been dying from heart disease at a higher rate than men.

I am a volunteer spokesperson for the American Heart Association. However, I didn't wait for permission to share with women about their risks of heart disease. I couldn't wait. I don't know how to wait. I wish I did. I wish I could learn to knit, enjoy reading novels, and drink tea with my girlfriends. Instead, I live with the need to communicate everything that I experienced during my grueling, miserably alone heart ordeal.

Each time I speak, I find that most women are stunned by what I have to say, and eager to see research that backs up the shocking news that heart disease, not breast cancer, is the number-one killer of American women.

Who knew? And yet women die from heart disease six times more than from breast cancer. Twice as many women die from heart disease as from all cancers put together! More women than men die of heart disease each year. But women receive only:

- 33% of the angioplasties, stents, and bypass surgeries that are performed;
- 28% of implantable defibrillators; and
- 36% of open-heart surgeries.

And women comprise only 25% of participants in all heart-related research studies (*Journal of the American Medical Association*, vol. 266, 1991, p. 559).

In reality, I don't feel like a survivor of heart disease. Why not? Because heart disease doesn't go away. I survived the 1994 Northridge earthquake. When I was pregnant in the summer of 1978, I survived climbing the Desert Fortress Masada, overlooking the Dead Sea in Israel. The term "survivor" represents what I've lived through or persisted through, like plants survive the frost. Yes, I did survive what I experienced in June 2003. I am surviving — and actually learning to thrive with heart disease. I'm thankful to wake up every morning, and every day I try to make right choices.

I am a mother, a grandmother, a daughter, and a sister. I have successfully climbed the corporate ladder and have had the same ladder pulled out from under me. I am writing this book for:

— all the women I speak to, 90% of whom do not know or have not accepted that heart disease is our number-one killer.

— the women who believe that ignorance is bliss.

— the women who haven't heard the news that it *does* matter if your father, uncle, or grandmother had heart disease.

— the women who believe that women — especially young women — are not supposed to have heart disease.

— the women who have given up listening to their bodies because every time they go to the doctor it's dismissed as neurosis.

— the women who simply don't want to be bothered, who are determined not to travel down the road I want to take them.

This book puts a face to women's heart disease: mine. I am your neighbor, your sister, your co-worker, the woman next to you panting on the treadmill — and yes, that's me you see Saturday morning at the grocery store. I am not a doctor, and this book isn't a medical guide, nor is it another book filled only with facts, figures, and data. It's an honest story by someone who has lived through the trials of life and matters of the heart. Women relate to women, especially a woman who shares what's happening deep within her chest. Once you see my heart, your own heart will become clearer. You will find the power to stand eye-to-eye with your doctor and represent yourself truly.

I mean to empower and encourage you to take better care of yourself, to be your own advocate and trust your God-given intuition.

Trust yourself. Love yourself. This is the heart of my message to you.

Chapter 1

Young and a Woman

June 8, 2003. I had looked forward to the Book Expo for months. I knew it would be the catalyst of big things to come. I planned to attend seminars the first day, where I would learn the mysteries of book writing, marketing, and publicity. Surely I would be able to meet some influential people.

But I wasn't emotionally prepared to see the famous writers I had envisioned standing right in front of me, walking among us mere mortals. I sat in awe of the hundreds of other attendees' boldness and determination to greet and meet all those writers and editors. At least I have tomorrow, I comforted myself. The next day was going to be an opportunity to visit all the exhibits; supposedly the speakers would be accessible.

The next morning my friend and I proudly wore our badges, ready to attack the convention center with gusto. After our first lap around the exhibits I was feeling exhausted, but I didn't say anything. As we approached our second lap, we had to climb some stairs. My friend said, "You don't look so good. Do you feel okay?" I was in a great mood, but my legs were weak, and I thought that maybe eating lunch away from the commotion would help me feel better. I opted to leave. It was what you call fatigue — though I had yet to recognize it as such.

Looking back from that moment, I realize now that for several weeks my right hand had been feeling numb, mostly at night. It was a pins-and-needles sensation that made holding a cold glass of iced tea feel great. Sometimes my chest would feel rather heavy, but I attributed that to a long day, maybe a glass of wine, or eating dinner too late. The hand-tingling bothered me enough to research carpal tunnel syndrome and mention it to my boss. I didn't want to be one of those employees who showed up for work one day with a brace on my wrist, and next thing I'm out on disability. Plus a brace wouldn't go well with most of my outfits.

For two solid weeks my hand had bothered me enough to mention it daily. I also had a little secret. The left side of my head, just over the ear, would get a tingling sensation that lasted about three seconds and then made me sneeze. Truly unusual, and I thought about seeing my doctor. But then I thought, how stupid would I feel, sitting down in the chair and saying, "Well, doctor, my head tingles and then I sneeze."

Ten years earlier — with the world's most rundown body, serious depression, pleurisy, and a collapsed stomach — I had been diagnosed with liver disease. The disease was horrific, and so was the treatment proposed to me. In 1993-94 I had been given the great honor and privilege of being selected to be what every woman dreams about. To be on the cover of a fashion magazine? No. To be honored for great achievements for my work in the inner city? No. For the seminars I had done in honor of women's causes? No. To be a human guinea pig for UCI Liver Research Department? That's it!

Told that there was only a slim chance of recovery, I had been selected to be one of 370 patients in the United States to try an experimental drug therapy program for liver disease: Interferon alfa-2A. My odds, I was told: a 50% chance of survival after 10 years with treatment, and less without. They chose me because I was "young and a woman." Flattering? Hardly. In fact, it was downright shocking. Sadly, at 37 years of age, too sick to walk up the stairs in my home — not to mention being faced with the prospect of not being there for my three daughters and my husband — I gave in to despair. In addition, the information the doctors gave me detailing the side effects of the experimental dosages were even more frightening than the disease itself.

After much thought, and with no other good options, I agreed to the treatment. I had nothing to lose and a lot to live for. For the next six months I found different areas in my home to lie in for hours upon hours, basically comatose. My three beautiful daughters and my unshakable husband and partner for life would see nothing more than a limp, lifeless, yellow body — except, of course, for my bouts of anger, depression, and nausea.

After all that, I awoke in March of 1994 completely well! Truly a miracle. No medications, no relapse, a clean bill of health. If you have watched "Touched by an Angel," you know that miracles usually require some action on the part of the human. My miracle was aided by injecting a massive dose of not-yet-FDA-approved drugs directly into my own thigh every other day. Many times I wanted to inject the medicine into someone else's thigh. And just as often I simply wanted to poke somebody else with the needle.

In 2003 my family threw a huge birthday celebration for me. The celebration marked 10 years from a time that I still have trouble believing ever existed. When you go through a sickness of that magnitude, it's often easier to believe it never happened. Yes, I can take out the pictures of the golden Lois, a yellow, almost-bronze Lois, so skinny that my nose and shinbones were my most prominent features. It's almost too intense to revisit. Maybe they just told me I was sick so they'd have a statistic on someone getting well. Maybe. . .

So with all that well in my past, the numbness in my hand, the annoying sneezing throughout the day, and the tingling in my brain prompted me to visit the doctor — the same doctor who had followed my saga for the previous 10 years. I figured if there was anyone I could share these weird symptoms with, he'd be the one.

The next Wednesday, however, when I was actually sitting in front of him, I told him only about the symptoms in my right hand. He agreed that it sounded like carpal tunnel syndrome and referred me to an orthopedist. But he also suggested having an electrocardiogram (EKG) before I left his office. An EKG takes longer to set up than to actually perform, so by the time I buttoned my shirt I heard the nurse tell the doctor the results were abnormal. He scheduled two additional heart tests: a 24-hour Holter monitor and an echocardiography.

Upon hearing that my EKG was abnormal, I didn't jump with joy, but I figured it was a result of my having rushed there from work without eating breakfast or lunch. No big deal. I told the nurse that I'd be back on Friday to get hooked up to the 24-hour Holter monitor. That way I could wear it over the weekend in the privacy of my own home. Returning to work with what looks like a transistor radio attached to a fanny pack just didn't work for me.

Plus, let's face it, I didn't take the time to let that abnormal EKG reading sink into my overproductive mind. Could it be something serious? Nah. No way.

That night we had a business meeting and dinner planned. While waiting my turn to speak, I became really anxious; I started biting my nails to the bone and couldn't calm myself down. I thought a piece of chocolate cake would help. I never eat cake, I thought, so it would do the trick. It didn't. When I got home that night, I stayed up talking to my youngest daughter a little later than normal. I remember telling her that my heart hurt.

The next day I stayed home from work. I couldn't say exactly why — just that I felt extra sensitive and couldn't imagine being around a lot of people. The same thing happened on Friday — highly unusual for me. I had left my laptop open at work with unfinished spreadsheets neatly displayed, and I had left personal letters, without stamps, waiting to be mailed. Again, not like me.

After a short trip to the store, I could no longer dismiss the feelings of radiating pain. Heartbeats of pain. My chest felt heavy. It felt like a pair of really big hands was squeezing my chest, like an elephant's enormous feet were pressing outward on my chest.

My husband arrived home at 8:30 p.m., and before he got comfortable I told him, "This might sound weird, but I think I need to go to the hospital. My chest and back are really bothering me." I hadn't fully convinced myself that something was the matter, and so I wasn't dressed to leave. I thought he'd say something comforting and I'd feel all better. Instead, he said, "Why don't you put your tennis shoes on and we'll go over to the hospital. It's not late, and this way we'll both sleep better tonight."

> With tears squeezing out of the corners of my eyes, I looked at my husband and asked, "What in the world is happening to me?"

If he had said, "No, let's wait, and you'll feel better in the morning," it wouldn't have made him uncaring. But it could have made him a widower. As it happened, I didn't don a running suit and sneakers, as he suggested. In my rush to leave, I threw on the first dress I found in my closet. A red dress, much worn and comfortable, like a good friend. Only much later did the irony of my choice of garments dawn on me. A red dress. . .

We chose the small community hospital down the street rather than the large hospital a few miles away. No big deal — it was just for our peace of mind. As it turned out, though, it *was* a big deal. Later that evening the kind ER doctor administered nitroglycerin and said, "I'm glad you're here." With tears squeezing out of the corners of my eyes, I looked at my husband and asked, "What in the world is happening to me?"

Nitroglycerin is given to prevent and treat angina pectoris (suffocating chest pain). This condition occurs when the coronary arteries become constricted and are not able to carry sufficient oxygen to the heart muscle. Nitroglycerin improves oxygen flow by relaxing the walls of arteries and veins, thus allowing them to dilate. In my situation, rather than feeling like each breath had a bag of cement attached to it, I felt I could breathe and become completely aware of the excruciating headache caused by the nitroglycerin.

The standard blood tests they take at such times as this show only if you've had a heart attack, not (and this is important) if the heart attack is actually in progress. About an hour or so later, the blood tests showed that I had not had a heart attack. We tried to relax. As a precaution, they kept me overnight in the hospital and arranged for a cardiologist to see me the next day, Saturday. That morning he visited my room, and again I was told, "You're young and a woman. I think it's probably acid reflux, and women have abnormal EKG's. Let's schedule a stress/echo test this week. Since it's the weekend, you'll feel better at home."

Okay, here's another secret. I didn't believe for one minute that I had acid reflux. I've *had* acid reflux and been on the "purple pill"; it wasn't the same feeling at all. But did I say anything? No. Women have abnormal EKG's? That's news to me — especially with *my* personal health history. But it's easy to feel stupid when someone in a position of authority is telling you something you know is wrong, and I felt stupid. I'm writing this so *you* won't be stupid.

On Sunday my daughter and I went to have our nails done. While watching the polish being applied, I thought to myself, "I'm probably having the worst acid reflux I've ever had." My back hurt about 10 times worse than it had on Friday night, and I felt lightheaded. I asked my daughter to drive, and she replied, "Mom, my nails are wet, too." However, I didn't want to go home, so she drove me to the "big hospital" a few miles away.

In the emergency room, we had to play musical chairs with all the other people and their children. "I'm out of here," I said finally. "This is dumb. I'm not staying. I'm fine." My daughter said, "Mom, please tell the lady at the desk you're having a heart attack! Why is that so difficult?" I casually walked up to the apathetic woman behind the desk and said, "My chest is really hurting, and I'm a little anxious about waiting too long." With great lethargy she assured me when the nurse finished with her current patient they'd call my name. Yippee. Back to musical chairs.

The next hour brought EKG's and blood tests, all ordered by a comforting young female physician. She did *not* tell me, "You're young and a woman." She asked about all my symptoms, my family history, and what had happened on Friday night at the emergency room at the other hospital. She also said there was no good reason why my EKG's should have been abnormal. *This* "abnormal" EKG made my third one.

As hospital protocol would have it, though, another doctor had to see me also. This guy would have topped the list of the 20 most undesirable people you'd like to never have a drink with, let alone give you a critical diagnosis. He started ugly and got worse.

"You're young and a woman," he said in his most patronizing bedside manner. "Did you think of taking Pepcid? Women have abnormal EKG's." Wait, get this, it got worse. He continued, "If I had to bet my last nickel, I'd put it on your stomach. And I disagree with my colleague. You shouldn't stay overnight."

My husband and I actually heard him arguing with the first doctor. So, over great reluctance on the part of Dr. "You've Got Indigestion," I stayed in the hospital that night. I was assured that I'd be home by noon the next day, right after the stress test. And make no mistake: His assurance was arrogance that he was right and I was wrong.

Side joke: What's the difference between God and a cardiologist? God knows he's not a cardiologist.

Monday afternoon, after another half dozen "young and a woman" comments, the cardiac nurse assigned to me told me that I'd be staying another night. My stress test showed some "finding." Tuesday morning, the cardiologist stopped by briefly to inform me, again, that women have abnormal EKG's and that he didn't think the "finding" amounted to much. He scheduled an angiogram for the next day, Wednesday.

Now the stress test, it turns out, is only 85% accurate, but the angiogram is 100% accurate. And my angiogram couldn't be scheduled for Tuesday because the cardiologist was busy with other patients. Oh boy — another day in the hospital, knowing that my chest pain was relieved only by the nitroglycerin patches which I had worn since Friday. To make my stay even more pleasant, I received injections in the stomach with some type of blood thinner that burned. Being hooked up to a heart monitor and having an IV drip wasn't too bad. The most fun part was having my fluids measured; every time I wanted to make the trip to the bathroom, I'd have to ask my roommate if she had left her potty in there. Did I mention that she was pushing 70, and didn't have a lot of sympathy or warm feelings for me? The funny thing is that she went home in perfect health and I went to intensive care. Actually, that isn't funny.

Finally, after an eternity of Dr. Phil and reality TV, Wednesday arrived. Time for the angiogram. I knew a tube would be inserted into my groin and jimmied all the way up into my heart. We would all see on the monitors what was really happening inside the heart of this "young woman." Except this "young woman" was shaking so intensely that they administered more sedation and I missed my big show on the monitor. But I do remember being whisked through hallways I hadn't seen before and taken to a very private room, where two nurses attached me to every machine known to mankind. By golly, finally I'd made it to intensive care! Suddenly I had become a very important "young woman."

The aides who rushed me to the ICU gave me more information about my condition than anyone else had. They told me that my left artery was blocked, and also that I wouldn't remember much of what they were explaining. Flat on my back, groggy, with my right leg tied down and a plug in my groin, it seemed time to become a bit concerned. To make matters worse, ICU doesn't allow phone calls. Talking to my parents in Oregon wasn't going to be easy.

The diagnosis: Coronary Artery Disease (CAD). To add to that diagnosis, the cardiologist explained I have small vessel disease. (Couldn't he have said "small thigh disease" instead? "Lois, I have to tell you that no matter what you do for the rest of your life — no exercise and a high-fat, high-carb, sugar-packed diet — your thighs will never get any bigger." Heaven!) No, instead he told me that I have a compromised circulatory system, sometimes referred to as "small vessel disease," in which arteries, veins, and capillaries are unusually small.

The "normal" angiogram procedure would be a cardiac catheter — a long, thin, soft tube inserted through an artery into the heart, allowing the doctors to immediately know if a blockage exists. (A quick lesson on catheters: A Foley catheter is a thin, sterile tube inserted into your bladder to drain urine. Because it can be left in place in the bladder for some time, it is also called an in-dwelling catheter.) The reason I'm relating this tidbit of information is because I didn't understand, while in intensive care, that they referred to my in-dwelling body fluid relief tube as a "Foley." What did I know? The reality was that — whatever they were called — I had one catheter up my groin and another in my bladder. The names didn't seem terribly important just then.

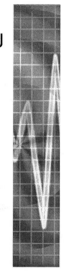

Only *you* know if you are experiencing something unique to your normal health patterns. Listen to what your body is telling you!

Now, back to my heart. If arterial blockage exists, then open heart surgery is performed, or a stent is immediately inserted into the blocked artery or arteries, the catheter removed, and the incision closed. (A stent, by the way, is simply a tube inserted into a blocked artery to hold it open so that blood can flow freely.) In my case, the doctors discovered that my left descending artery (often referred to as the "widow maker") was 75% blocked. But, since I was "young and a woman" there was no stent readily available for my size artery. Therefore, they had to leave the artery in my groin open until the next day. Highly dangerous, I discovered later.

The following morning, back down I went on the flat metal bed, knocked out cold, while a drug-eluting coronary stent (one that releases a drug gradually over time) was positioned in my troublesome artery. Then a special stitch and a plug made of collagen were placed in the incision. I'd like to mention that if I were going to have collagen inserted into my body, my first choice would be my lips, perhaps around the eye area, but not my groin. I must say, however, that my right groin has never looked so ample. What a comfort.

Once I regained consciousness, I felt as if I had been given a shot of pure oxygen. I had no idea how much better breathing could be! Opening up my artery relieved all those years of yawning uncontrollably at the gym, yawning to the point of embarrassment.

Why am I telling you this?

We women need to pay attention to our bodies. If I had not listened to my body and sheepishly returned to ER, but nonetheless returned, I would not be writing and speaking about heart disease today. Only *you* know if you are experiencing something unique to your normal health patterns. Listen to what your body is telling you!

Heart disease is for the rest of my life. Genetics play the largest role in my fight with heart disease, but that doesn't excuse me from doing my part.

Allow me to slip out of my puke-green hospital attire and into my favorite old sweatsuit. Let me grab my discharge papers and the handful of brochures that tell me more about coronary artery disease than I ever wanted to know, and slide gingerly, almost gracefully, like a bird with a damaged wing, a butterfly bursting out of its cocoon, into the wheelchair that would take me curbside. From that point I will cautiously place my body into the vehicle that will transport me back to a place I left six days earlier.

With one major difference: This time, when I sit in my living room, I won't be wondering about the elephant that is sitting on my chest. Instead I will be assessing the damage that elephant has done to my husband, my daughters — and my future.

Chapter 2

Living with an Elephant

Whenever I'm asked what a heart attack feels like, I reply: "like an elephant sitting on my chest." (Let me emphasize that my own elephant sat on my back first, making it hard to steer a car, sit up straight, or shrug it off as a sore muscle from working out. Later I found out that the phenomenon of the pain beginning in the back, and then moving to the chest, is atypical for men, but typical for women.) Often the elephant seemed to have brought his whole family to visit. And that elephant and his family had caused me to return to the emergency room for a second time in less than 24 hours.

Little wonder that the people in my life felt some of the elephant's enormous weight too. *You* try to conceal massive amounts of pain from those closest to you. No matter how much you want to protect your loved ones, the symptoms — unrelenting pain in the chest, shots of electrifying impulses radiating between your shoulder blades — are bound to be apparent. They certainly were when heart disease attacked my dad — and now it was my turn.

Even before I was diagnosed with heart disease, I was well aware (thanks to my family history) of how heart disease affects one's life and one's family. I even bought a book called *The Complete Idiot's Guide to a Happy, Healthy Heart*. Did I read it? No, I was an idiot and waited until I had heart disease to pull it off my bookshelf.

Since being diagnosed with coronary artery disease (CAD), I've learned so much about sudden cardiac arrest — the hard way. The most common underlying reason for sudden death from cardiac arrest is fatty buildups in the arteries that block blood supply to the heart muscle. About 335,000 people a year die of coronary heart disease without being hospitalized or admitted to an emergency room — more than 930 deaths every day. That's about half of all deaths from heart disease. And the victims may not even know that they have heart problems!

But now I knew that simple, inescapable fact all too well, and my life would never be the same. I felt as if the elephant had climbed off my chest, only to take a permanent seat in my living room. Everywhere I looked I felt his presence. It's not a long drive from the hospital to our home; that day, however, the trip seemed much longer than usual. Only a few days had passed since my first visit to the emergency room, but I felt as if months had gone by. I felt like an entirely different person — fragile, tentative, unspeakably anxious to get home to my husband and my children, though I carried a new burden: the secret anxiety of a wife and mother about their well-being.

Please try to imagine yourself in my place. As mothers, we have so very many things that we can reflect on and feel good about. But there's a dark side of motherhood also: the nurturer's fears for those little beings whom she has ushered into this world. Mothers never, ever cease feeling responsible; they never outgrow the urge to protect. And now, suddenly, my ongoing ability to protect my daughters had been placed at terrible risk. I am one woman speaking on behalf of the six million women who live with heart disease. I have a voice to speak, arms to hug my family, eyes to see my surroundings, and a mind to see my future. A half million women each year do not have these same opportunities.

> **I am one woman speaking on behalf of the six million women who live with heart disease. I have a voice to speak, arms to hug my family, eyes to see my surroundings, and a mind to see my future. A half million women each year do not have these same opportunities.**

My oldest daughter Bethany, who was expecting our first grandchild, arrived the next day. Just a week after her wedding, she and her husband had packed up and moved to northern California, where he had been hired as a firefighter. A great opportunity, sure, but it meant she would be away from her sisters, all two years apart and still so involved in each other's daily lives.

Bethany's move meant that I wouldn't be able to be with her as her baby grew inside of her, as she experienced pregnancy for the first time. She loves to be with family 24 hours a day. I can't think of a time when she ever asked to be alone. If she could have a nonstop slumber party, it would be fine with her. Even now she hates the dark. She's still the little girl who wants someone to go before her and turn on the lights.

I couldn't imagine upsetting her with bad news, especially now that she was carrying my first grandchild. She wasn't able to be with me at all while I was in the hospital. More important to me as her mother, I wasn't able to comfort her about the fact that I was in the hospital. Nurturers of the world — *mothers* of the world — understand what I mean here. When Bethany asked about my heart problems, I would turn the subject back to her.

Again, please understand my deepest fear. I knew that my father's heart condition had been passed along to me, his only daughter. How could I not think about the possibility that my own dear daughters — or even my unborn grandchild — might be carrying the seeds of the same terrible condition? Frightening beyond words, and yet not something that I felt able to communicate to them, or protect them from.

My middle daughter, Cortney, came immediately to the hospital. As she entered my room I could see the stress on her face. It was obvious she had been crying. Of the three girls, Cortney is most like me. She stayed with me for most of every day while I was hospitalized, sitting for hours without complaining. She was (and is) a great comfort to me. And being the middle child isn't an easy role. You're not the oldest, with the privileges of that position; you're not the youngest, and the adored baby of the family. You're stuck in the middle. I love all three of my girls, but if I had a nickel for every time Cortney said I didn't love her as much as the other two, I could retire tomorrow.

In a crisis, though, Cortney is the one to lean on. She likes being in charge. She eased her pain, and her fears about me, by dishing out assignments and keeping her father in line. She made all the necessary calls to my parents, brothers, and other family members. My husband Tim still talks about what a drill sergeant she was. She even had to feed me when I was in intensive care, when I wasn't allowed to sit up because the artery in my groin was open. Now I ask you, mothers of any age, at what point in this life do we want our own children to feed us with a spoon? Right. *Never.*

Fortunately, my youngest daughter Michal wasn't home when I went to the emergency room. She was away at college, and I was thankful for that. It hadn't been that long since we were in the same emergency room with her, after she suffered a serious biking accident. Her being absent spared us all, at least, the added trauma of revisiting that event with her. Plus, she is such a nurturer (I wonder where she gets that trait?) that I had to keep her a little in the dark so that she wouldn't ditch classes to look after her mom.

So as you can see, I hope, with my three beautiful girls so deeply intertwined in my heart, I wanted desperately to believe that the elephant on my chest had only been acute indigestion. Unfortunately, it wasn't indigestion, and I could no longer pretend.

Before I left the hospital I was given a few gifts: a list of medications and suggestions for revising my lifestyle. What did I do? Cried, of course — with no waterproof mascara handy. Wherever I turned, in every part of my life, there was that elephant again. I needed to come up with a game plan. How do you get an elephant out of your life? Eat it? Scare it away? Right now, though, I was the one who was scared.

It was Friday afternoon — exactly one week from the day I went to the emergency room. I sat in my living room, in the same exact spot where I had sat seven days before. The intense back pain that had radiated into my chest was gone. Instead I was filled with weakness, confusion, and some disbelief. The elephant wasn't on my chest, but I could feel his presence in my house. Perhaps he's hiding around the corner, I thought, and will appear just when I relax. Or maybe he was lurking upstairs, ready to rest one of his enormous feet on my chest when I lay down on my bed.

On the coffee table in front of me was my daunting assortment of daily medications. I separated the pills neatly into three separate sections: Morning, Evening, and Bedtime. There I sat, alone in my family room, or almost alone: just me, my new pills, and the elephant.

I knew one thing for sure: I needed desperately to understand what coronary artery disease was all about, and how having CAD would affect my life. (For starters, since June 2003 I have purchased every book available on Amazon.com about women's heart disease.) I've always prided myself on my organizational skills. Ask me to organize something, and I'm there with colored folders, markers, Post-it notes, and pens. In my working life, any job I'd applied for had been mine for the taking; sometimes I'd had to choose between two jobs. Now I needed to use these same organizational skills to reorganize my life around taking pills, preparing food differently, and making sure I got to cardio rehabilitation three times a week.

As I pondered the project at hand (let's label the folder Lois Trader's New Life), which included accepting the need to choke down a wad of pills every day, I realized that I had a much bigger mission. No diagnosis, even heart disease, would allow me to ignore this. (Try not to snicker at what I'm about to say, please. It tells you a lot about me.) I had determined earlier — pre-heart attack — to buy a new recliner for my husband's birthday and Father's Day. I had arrived home from the hospital on June 15. My husband's birthday is June 16, and June 17 was Father's Day. June 18 was our anniversary — 26 years together. My course of action was clear. My heart was *not* going to stop me.

So, on my second day home, my daughter Bethany drove me to three different furniture stores until I found the perfect recliner. At the first store I heard the salesman say to Bethany, "Your mom looks like she doesn't feel well." If you're a bit amazed that I didn't even consider purchasing the chair another time, well, so am I — now. At the time, however, I behaved as if nothing unusual had happened in my life; I even organized the delivery of the precious recliner — surprise delivery, by the way, which involved a neighbor who was entirely oblivious that anything untoward had taken place in the Trader household. I'm a woman, after all, and matriarch of the family; I didn't want to disappoint.

The next Monday my husband returned to work. Bethany and her husband headed back up north; Cortney had work and college; and Michal lived on campus. I was home alone — just me and that elephant. I hope you can comprehend the state of mind of someone who has suffered a heart attack: As far as we know, that elephant can reappear at any minute. Medicines or no medicines, you don't feel safe.

The coffee table was still covered with my new prescriptions. Nothing had moved. Even with the arrival of the recliner, the prescriptions were left in place — a part of my life décor. Well, I put all the little pills in their slots, under each day of the week. My plan was to rely on these containers, to become acquainted with them, to learn to love them even (and perhaps to trade them in for more colorful ones).

But I was also hungry! No one was around to offer me a healthy sandwich. I would have loved a delicious tuna sandwich, with pickle relish and lots of alfalfa sprouts. I walked into the kitchen and read the labels on cans. I'd been warned that I must limit my intake of salt; though the calculations were new to me, it was apparent that a single can of tuna would be my quota for the day. Believe me, no one is ever prepared to find that one lonely can of tuna — once a mainstay for lunch — is no longer a friend. One can of tuna has 250 mg. of salt and an additional 30 mg. of cholesterol. Bye-bye, tuna! Chowing down on protein had always been a way of watching my weight, but a diet consisting mostly of protein wasn't displayed on the Heart Healthy pyramid. What to do? I gave up the idea and decided to check in with my employer.

Big mistake. Somehow I had thought that a heart attack might merit some time off to recuperate. Wrong. Instead I learned that my boss had decided it would be best if I didn't go on disability, and that I should work from home for a week or so, starting immediately. I wasn't consulted on that decision. Late that day she called. I had missed the important Denver trip, not to mention a full week of work. I felt sick and exhausted while she was talking, but I didn't tell her that. I didn't tell her that I should be left alone, not thinking about anything but getting well. A voice inside my head was trying to tell me, "Lois, this is not a good thing." I wasn't listening — yet.

The following weekend my boss insisted on taking me out for coffee. I felt as if she didn't believe that I was really ill and wanted to see herself. Maybe she blamed herself for hiring a person who turned out to be a dud. Less than six months on the job and I'd suffered a heart attack! What does that say about her judgment?

Here's the problem: You can't see heart disease. Oh, you could see that I looked tired and a little pale, but my hair was done and I had on makeup. Sure I found the time to brush on some mascara — I mean, I'm not dead!

When I returned to work I looked exactly like my old self. Heart disease isn't pretty, and during my hospital stay I *certainly* wasn't pretty. But after a week or two at home, I looked like the old Lois. I *wasn't* myself, though. I was a woman who, at age 47, had been told that she has coronary artery disease. A woman who on the outside inherited her mother's genes (I look younger than I am), but on the inside had inherited her father's genes (my arteries are 20 years older than I am). My outside appearance was now working against me. So was my need for acceptance.

> At work, I'm sure that I defied everyone's idea of what heart disease looks like. So, within a day, I was treated exactly the same. Worse, in fact, I had to prove I was worthy of my job, that I could do it, do it all.

At work, I'm sure that I defied everyone's idea of what heart disease looks like. So, within a day, I was treated exactly the same. Worse, in fact. I had to prove I was worthy of my job, that I could do it, do it all. I was given assignments galore. Crazy? Absolutely. I knew it wasn't healthy. Before my heart attack I drove 32 miles to work one way. Now I was told that I'd be supporting a new group located 55 miles away — and in downtown Los Angeles, at that. Insane.

What was going on? Was I supposed to quit? Was I supposed to go out on disability? I was stuck in all-day meetings, where no one stopped for lunch. Let's see, I'm supposed to be eating balanced, heart-healthy meals; I'm supposed to put aside my old ways that helped clog my arteries. I needed to eat fruits, vegetables, and grains — and *not* skip meals. Otherwise, I'd get too hungry and grab the first thing I saw instead of the correct foods. In addition, I was trying to adjust to my medications, and trying to figure out why the muscles in my calves were numb. Was it from sitting too long at meetings, or was it a side effect from the drugs?

There was that one day when my legs simply would not work. (I think it was a side effect from a new drug.) I knew my heart was fine and my head wasn't foggy, but I had to ask a friend to meet me at work and drive me to get something to eat. I was still learning all the new things that I needed to know and learning how to live with this disease — and here I was back at work, trying to look good and keep my salary.

Without a doubt, I had picked the wrong employer. I confess I knew that from the beginning. I took the job for a big pay increase, rather than staying in a healthy, fun working environment. Absolutely the wrong job for the new me, obviously.

I sensed that I was at a crossroads in my life. Never before had I felt so alone, though I was surrounded with people. I shared my concerns with my husband, who has been a rock for me — living through so much and having to be positive. But he too was challenged by our new situation. He was scared of losing his wife, scared that we had a huge mortgage and two daughters in college. We depended on my salary. He knew if he agreed with my concerns, I might be more likely to consider a change. In sickness and in health, he was being challenged.

I knew that Tim was also wondering if his wife would ever be normal again. Would I die prematurely as my father had? My dad always looked great on the outside; he was fit, played tennis, enjoyed swimming and boating. Tim saw our similarities, and I knew that, for all his light-hearted personality, he was deeply troubled. I could almost read his thoughts and fears: What if I had another heart attack? What if I were to become disabled? Would our insurance cover the hospital stay and all my new prescriptions? If I decided I couldn't work anymore, could we afford my medical bills?

I was questioning everything, from my very existence to my daily tasks, and Tim knew it. I knew he appreciated the fact that I was more focused on health and well-being. Certainly my former lifestyle had contributed to this early heart disease, after all. I found myself trying to reshape my life and discuss with him the emotional and psychological healing (not to mention the physical healing!) that lay ahead. I needed to know that he understood my renewed appreciation for the fragility of life. I wanted understanding and compassion for how difficult and painful it can be to live with the elephant of heart disease. I wanted to be hugged more — just hugged. I wanted him and my daughters — and everyone! — to understand my mood swings, tears, fears (for me and for them), and confusion. Little things meant so much to me. When Tim gave me a brightly colored coffee cup to cheer up my mornings, it was so sweet and made me feel so good that — well, I cried, of course.

I wanted everyone to understand that the elephant wasn't sitting on my chest any longer, but I could see him everywhere I looked; learning to live with the elephant's constant presence was one of the very hardest lessons that I had to learn. When I sat

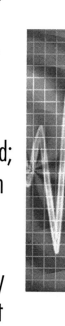

> I wanted everyone to understand that the elephant wasn't sitting on my chest any longer, but I could see him everywhere I looked; learning to live with the elephant's constant presence was one of the very hardest lessons that I had to learn.

in the family room, I saw the elephant. When I went to work, there he was. He didn't seem to be leaving simply because I had survived his last visit.

At about that same time, my cardiologist signed me up for cardio rehabilitation. To get there, I had to leave work early three days a week so I could make it to the last class of the day. To me, this was just one more reminder that I had heart disease, but all my co-workers and my boss saw was me walking out the door early. The novelty wore off quickly. The first day, after I changed clothes in the company bathroom, I heard cries of "Oh, your sweatsuit is so cute!" By the second week the comments had changed to "Where are you going, Lois?" — though they knew where I was going.

Six full weeks of cardio rehab was not going to be a solid career move, I realized. And to my shame, I actually didn't graduate from rehab. I wanted to get the certificate and the applause for completing the course, but I just couldn't keep the appointments. It was becoming increasingly clear that I was keeping my job at the expense of my health — at the expense of my heart.

Remember, I was being forced to drive into downtown Los Angeles every day, and there was no way of making it back to the rehab center by 3:00. I was aware that my boss knew that fact very well. I would sigh loudly and clearly when 3:00 came and went. I tried to make believe that the long walk to my car was sufficient exercise, but I was kidding myself.

In the beginning, though — before the conflicts at work won out — I was kind of energized to join the rehab group. I was sure that I'd learn a lot. I thought I might even meet other women with heart disease, and we could become friends. Until that time the only stories I'd heard had been about someone's mother or father with heart disease — people 20 or 30 years older than me. As it turned out, however, all my rehab teammates were older (much older) men. Not another woman, of any age, in sight.

Unfortunately, that rehab experience made me feel considerably more alone in my fight with heart disease. It's tough when even the other heart patients don't believe that you have heart disease. The old boys weren't buying it, and I didn't have the energy to share what I'd been through.

I thought it would be cool and stylish to sport a ribbon to rehab — a ribbon that represented women's heart disease. After all, I might as well identify with my disease; think of it as "Embracing the Elephant." I wanted to purchase one from a site on the Internet, but searched to no avail. Could it be that the number-one killer of American women is ribbonless? I found sites where I could purchase a ribbon representing countless different diseases. I discover, for instance, that I could purchase a ribbon for colon cancer (brown, no less), or a pink and blue ribbon allowing men to show that they too have breast cancer.

Let me help you understand my eagerness to shout to the world my awareness of the dangers of heart disease. Before my heart attack, my top-priority concern had been breast cancer (as is true of so many women). So when I went to the gym I would wear my New Balance sneakers with the pink ribbon embroidered on the tongue. Underneath my sweat suit would be my Wacoal bra (The Awareness Bra) with yet another embroidered pink ribbon. This bra actually comes with a tiny brochure that tells you how to self-examine your breasts. While reading *Self* magazine on the treadmill, I was reminded (over 15 times) through articles and advertisements that I needed to be aware of breast cancer. When I got home, I'd grab a container of Yoplait yogurt, knowing that by merely popping open the lid, I was supporting breast cancer research. After walking on the treadmill, my feet would be tired from so I'd slip on my Karen Neuburger comfy socks, again with the cute pink ribbon. Then I'd relax with a cup of coffee using my $25 limited-edition pink-ribbon coffee mug purchased from "The View's" website. Finally, in my bathroom you'd find nothing but Quilted Northern toilet paper, a proud sponsor of the Susan G. Komen Breast Cancer Foundation Race for the Cure Series.

Whew. But no ribbon for heart disease? I did learn that the American Heart Association has a program called "Go Red." All the women in the pictures wore a "Red Dress Pin," to identify women with our number-one killer. I purchased one immediately and proudly wore it to my first appointment at cardio rehab.

I knew that cardio rehabilitation was terribly important, but I was terrified about having back pain again. Who knew what might trigger it? Not me, that's for sure. Might another artery become clogged next time? What if the one with the stent implanted in it were to re-close? What would *that* feel like? One major function of cardio rehab is to help lower the patient's anxiety level about their disease and its effects on their everyday life. Rehab helps the patient create a routine where they can accept and realize that they won't die if they jog slowly on a treadmill, calmly row the rowing machine, and ride the bike for 10 minutes or so.

Early on, one of the rehab nurses showed me how to hook myself up to a portable EKG machine. First, clean off four areas around your chest. Second, stick the little white patches with the snap on those shiny clean areas. Third, walk over and grab a fanny pack and slip the portable EKG into it. The portable unit has four wires, each with a different color at the end; each wire attaches to the correct patch on your body (That in itself was a challenge for me. They should have colored the patches to match the wires, right? But no.) Tightening your fanny pack so you can exercise without the portable EKG falling out turns it into a charming accessory. One demonstration per heart patient and you're deemed an expert and must do it alone. Each time I arrived,

I tried to find an area around the corner to fumble with my new sticky electro-friend, afraid that baring my upper torso might set off a chain reaction of arrhythmia within the group.

The truth of the matter was that I had not yet gotten my arms around the fact that I had heart disease. Oozing with denial, I watched the nurses intently as they sat in front of the monitors that displayed our heart waves. I knew every time one of the nurses winced that it had to be because of my heart's abnormal beats.

> The truth of the matter was that I had not yet gotten my arms around the fact that I had heart disease.

If I were in charge of cardio rehabilitation, I would be sure that the first class dealt with what women are going through, helping us understand that we are not little men — we are women. I can't say exactly what I needed at that time, but I never quite got into the groove of the rehab classes. The weekly classes ranged from nutrition and stress management to discussing shopping lists and cooking differently. All the classes are undoubtedly important, but I would have added one dedicated solely to the depression one experiences following a heart attack. The thought of someone touching your heart, going anywhere near that precious organ, keeps you up at night. Fear of dying after a heart event is common! I wish I'd heard this kind of information sooner.

I cried a lot — not at rehab, though. There I made sure I looked good, was on time, and smiled on cue. I also made sure not to become too chatty with any of my teammates, since I didn't need any new male friends.

In the middle of all this disruption and terrible indecision, Bethany called me to say that when she got up from the couch she felt like she had gone to the bathroom. I asked her if the water still running down her legs. It was. I replied, "Call your husband and get to the hospital as soon as possible. Your water broke." She was seven months pregnant. I managed (I think) to sound calm.

So there was my dear Bethany going into premature labor, four hours away. Couple that with the news from my cardiologist, who was demanding that I leave my job and elect to go out on disability. None of my tests had shown improvement, he said. Here were two billboard-sized signs shouting at me: Change, Lois! Change! Plus, the signs told me, changing meant more than going to cardio rehab. It meant mental, emotional, and physical change — *life* rehab.

I know that getting upset is unhealthy for me. They told me in the class about stress. And I hadn't learned how to control it yet? Come on, I'm barely out of the hospital! Anyway, hadn't I read somewhere that we're supposed to get a grace period from stress? Probably the same place where I read "Only one sickness per human in a lifetime." I read it in my dreams on a lacy piece of paper that floats around and eventually blows away.

Surprisingly (to me, at least), leaving my job turned out to be easy. I didn't have the guts to call my boss directly. I sent her a fax — from my doctor's office, no less. Several months later I received a note telling me that my position was no longer needed.

Leaving for Fresno to meet my daughter at the hospital couldn't be done through a fax. Getting my other daughters together, my husband off work, packing up and starting our four-hour drive north wasn't easy. But we had to be there for her.

On our frantic drive to be with Bethany during her labor, I tried to sort out the last few months of my life. I tried to imagine how I'm going to get it together. How am I going to create a new life for myself, and for my family? I have to embrace this elephant — learn to love him (and even his family). And I've definitely got to quit crying.

I know that my cardiologist isn't a therapist, but I realize it's time that I admit to him how depressed I am. He's worried about my stress. We've talked about my work. He hasn't been happy with my blood tests, even questioning whether or not I was taking my prescriptions. If he knew me better, he'd know that's a really dumb question. Of course, I'm taking my prescriptions. Not missing a dose.

I determined that as soon as we get through this time with my daughter I would make an appointment with my cardiologist with the plan that I would discuss the elephant. Perhaps he could explain to me how to get rid of an elephant. . .

Chapter 3

Going Back in Time

The beginning of November 2003 — five months since the day I came home from the hospital. Every area of my life has been turned upside down. Time to get up the nerve to talk to my doctor about my depression.

Really, it shouldn't be too difficult. I mean, every time he's seen me since the hospital I'm about a second away from tears. With the slightest prompting I cry. I cried when my office manager asked me how I was doing. I cried when I got on the scale. (Well, like a lot of women, I still cry about that.) I didn't understand why every time I got on the scale at his office I seemed to have gained two pounds. He didn't seem to worry, but I was beside myself. I knew my body was going through a major overhaul, reacting to my cold-turkey approach to stopping hormone replacement therapy, though that was my lot for now. I cried when I talked about my medication. I didn't understand why I had heart disease. I was worried that I would die young, worried that I wouldn't be there for my daughters. I cried and cried.

"I've never felt like this before," I cried to my doctor, "and I think it's your fault!" He laughed at that one, and so did I. So he started trying to explain things to me. Gently, sweetly, carefully, he suggested that I might think about seeing a psychiatrist. He started to mention anti-depressants and caught himself. I wish he would have stopped there, but seeing me cry so much, I think he wanted to say something that would help.

What he said next made me want to crawl under the covers and stay there the rest of my life. It also made me angry. A few hours later, I realized that he had been trying to help me make sense of my whole situation. Heart disease, my doctor said (and this is one of the very most important things anyone has ever said to me), doesn't start with the diagnosis.

"Lois," he told me, "whatever you did when you were in your twenties is why you have heart disease today." To grasp that fact, to accept responsibility for my own heart disease, overwhelmed me. I did pretty darned well in my twenties — or so I thought. Before I was married, I'd watch Mary Tyler Moore on Friday nights when my friends were out drinking and going to parties. My diet was healthy (except for the times when I'd finish the entire cake). So, what did I do in my twenties that caused my heart disease today? Since then my doctor has learned more about my condition and the genetics I inherited, but I found myself musing about the first few decades of my life.

> When I was five years old, my dad disappeared for a long time. I didn't understand then that he had been hospitalized with a massive heart attack. He was 37 years old.

I grew up in a typical All-American family — the youngest of four children, and the only girl. Being the youngest and a twin (my brother Donald beat me out of the womb by eight minutes) gave me power over my brothers and prominence in the hearts of my parents. From very early in my life, however, I remember being aware of my father's heart problems. I remember an incident when Donald and I were barely 5 years old. We were wrestling with our dad when he told us that he couldn't play any more because his back hurt. Then he disappeared for a long time after that. I didn't understand then that he had been hospitalized with a massive heart attack. He was 37 years old.

When I turned 17, my dad's heart really took precedence in our home. He had been in and out of the hospital with two open heart surgeries, and complications from both. My dad had congestive heart failure, and atherosclerosis throughout his body. (Atherosclerosis occurs when deposits of fatty substances — cholesterol, cellular waste products, calcium, and other substances — build up in the inner lining of an artery. This buildup is called plaque. Plaques can grow large enough to significantly impede blood flow through an artery. But most of the damage occurs when plaques become fragile and rupture. Plaques that rupture cause blood clots to form that can block blood flow or break off and travel to another part of the body. Blockage of a blood vessel that feeds the heart causes a heart attack. If a blood vessel that feeds the brain is blocked, the result is a stroke.)

Our family had to come to terms with the fact that my dad was not going to live a full span of years. I have distinct memories of that time in my life. Being the only girl made my trips to the hospital a greater responsibility because I wanted to be there with my mom. My dad was a tough little guy; he always put on a brave face in front of us. But sometimes I would walk into the living room and catch him with his hands on his chest, counting his heartbeats.

On the morning of my dad's second open heart surgery, we got the news that my grandmother — my mother's mother — had died. I wondered, as a young person would, if her passing was a sign that my father would die too. Sitting, waiting, praying to hear if my father had made it through his surgery became somewhat surreal. The overload of worry, sadness, and mourning cast an invisible cloud over us.

At about that same time, my oldest brother Richard, who was married and had a baby girl, moved four hours away, to Pismo Beach. The fact that he was six years older than I and lived far away put a natural distance between us. But I loved him a lot. He never betrayed my secrets and my trust in him; he was a kind, sweet brother who had often stepped in as my "knight in shining armor." Not seeing him as frequently, some of his comments confused me. Often he seemed so frustrated, though never angry. He was frustrated over having to conform at work and fit into a mold that in prior years he had been able to escape. Once married with a child, the days of working odd jobs, living close to and spending endless time at the beach, disappeared completely.

I have one especially vivid memory of the day he left my parents' home. Just before the door closed, he turned and asked me if he could take a certain plant that had belonged to our grandmother. Without hesitation, I told him no. He looked directly at me and replied, "Why don't you come visit my apartment sometime?" I nodded my head as if to say sure and then closed the door. Looking back now, I know he was trying to reach out to me.

My parents knew their time together might be limited, so they planned a grand vacation in Hawaii. I had no reason to be troubled. I loved the thought of them in Hawaii — relaxing, soaking up the sun, and spending precious time together. But the first night they were away I slept horribly. I racked my brain, as I tossed and turned, wondering what could possibly be so disturbing.

The next morning I was tired, but I got up early and drove to college. Still overwhelmed with inexplicable uneasiness, I turned my car around before class started and drove back home, to find my brother Peter's car in the driveway. Peter, three years older than I, lived 40 minutes away and it was early; I knew instantly that he wasn't there for a social call. Within minutes I learned that when I had denied my oldest brother's request for the plant and closed the door, it would be the last time I would ever see him. Richard had committed suicide.

My body turned to lead. My mind was numb, except for one thought: Surely my father would never be able to survive this catastrophe. How can any parent endure the news that their oldest child (or any child, for that matter) has taken his own life? The days following this awful news felt as if our whole family had been left hanging over a cliff. My parents returning from Hawaii, the funeral for my brother, his widow and baby girl, my two brothers, relatives, friends, co-workers — all became a blur that I tucked away in some remote part of my brain. What I do remember clearly was my father leaning on the pillar of our front porch, crying, and saying over and over, "This is so terrible."

After my brother's death, every weekend my parents drove to Huntington Beach to pick up his baby girl, their first grandchild. But a few months after his death, when they went to pick Danielle up, no one was there. Wherever they turned, whatever they did, they could not find out what happened to their granddaughter or her mother. It was one more deep cut in our already bleeding hearts. A bottomless hole started with that terrible chain of events, seemingly never to be filled.

Time continues on, with or without our permission. Days became weeks, weeks became months, and several years passed from the day of my brother's death. My dad grew weaker and would often

Emotional Health and Your Heart

Stephanie Buehler, MPW, PsyD, CST

Tears may be dried up —
But the heart, never.
— Marguerite de Valois

What makes a healthy heart? Certainly a healthful diet that includes Omega 3 fatty acids, regular exercise, adequate sleep, very moderate alcohol consumption, and no smoking. But did you realize that your emotional health is actually a better predictor of heart health than your other healthful habits?

Scientist William Harvey (1578-1657) noticed a connection between heart and emotional health as early as 1625. Early physician William Osler said that the typical heart disease patient is "a keen and ambitious man, the indicator of whose engine is always 'full speed ahead'." Of course, to any woman reading Osler's observation, it is clear that things have changed for our gender; today, heart disease is the leading cause of death for today's woman, who seems always on the go and buffeted by conflicting demands.

Even so, the connection between emotions and heart disease is somewhat poorly understood. Anger, depression, anxiety, loneliness, and constant stress are the feelings that researchers have identified as putting women — and men — at risk for heart disease. Researchers and cardiologists Dr. Meyer S. Friedman and Dr. Ray Rosenman are credited with coining the term "Type A Personality" in the 1950's as basically an angry person who possesses three traits: free-floating hostility, impatience, and insecurity. "Trait anger" has also been associated with sudden cardiac death. People who score high on hostility scales more rapidly develop atherosclerosis. Perhaps most frightening of all, a Harvard study shows that 1 in 40 heart attack survivors experienced an "episode of anger" two hours before their heart attack.

For women, perhaps the most pertinent emotional experience associated with heart problems is depression, because depression is much more common for women than for men. A recent study demonstrated that patients who were depressed were three times more likely to die in the year following a heart attack. Also, women were twice as likely as men to develop depression after a heart attack.

Many people think of a depressed person as someone who is so deeply sad, hopeless, and lethargic that they are unable to function, but this is not so. There is also minor depression, in which a person has only a few symptoms, and dysthymia, a low-grade level of depression that continues for two years or longer. Depression can also occur after a major life-changing event such as a move. Finally, depression can be caused by a medical condition, such as multiple sclerosis or diabetes.

The problem with depression is that a woman who is depressed is less likely to notice her physical symptoms, or to do anything about them. It is well known that people who are depressed have trouble complying with their doctor's orders, including taking medication. A depressed woman is less likely to exercise or eat a healthful diet. All of these factors can lead to ill health, including heart disease.

Anxiety and chronic stress can also precipitate heart disease. Anxiety may be generalized — in other words, a person may worry and feel keyed up — much of the time, no matter what is happening, or it may be specific, as in a phobia of some kind. Obsessive-compulsive disorder, as well as its associated personality disorder, is also a manifestation of anxiety. Intense anxiety can trigger cardiac arrest as the heartbeat abruptly turns fast and uncoordinated. Fortunately, anxiety is one of the easiest

have to stop while taking a short walk to the corner. Congestive heart failure affected his every move. But my parents had always dreamed of a trip to Hong Kong. Against his cardiologist's objections, my dad insisted that they make the trip. So off to Hong Kong they went. I recall so vividly the night before they left: my dad playing with my baby girls, trying to get Cortney to smile.

The very first morning at breakfast, my mom told him that she could see his heartbeats through his shirt. Each breath was a labor for him. They quickly returned to their hotel room to call the doctor. Shortly thereafter, there in Hong Kong, my father was pronounced dead by an unfamiliar doctor as my mom stood by helplessly. He was 57 years old. My mom and I have discussed that day many times in detail. She knew my dad had passed away before the doctor arrived. Twenty years later, the story still makes my heart ache. I see my dad in dreams as if he were alive, and I awaken, amazed at how much I still miss him.

problems to treat, and for most people it can be managed without medication.

Chronic stress — work woes, financial problems, troubled marriage, caregiving, and even environmental stresses such as natural disasters — have also been linked with the development of heart disease. In my practice as a psychologist who teaches people ways to manage stress, I can say that the problem for most women is "must disease," as in "I must do everything — today! — and I must do it well, and I must please everyone." The only "must" in my mind is that women must learn to relax!

Further proof that anger, depression, anxiety, and stress lead to heart disease comes from the improvements that occur when these states are treated. The well-known Recurrent Coronary Prevention Project studied over 1,000 men and women who received routine medical care and group counseling about risk factors, or care plus group therapy to modify Type A traits. Those who attended group therapy had a whopping 44% reduction in second heart attacks. A similar longitudinal study demonstrated that not only do people who receive stress management have a significant reduction in second cardiac events, they also save an average of $1,228 in medical costs per year.

A whole-person approach to cardiac disease prevention is critical. When anyone recommends that you see a behavioral health specialist — a mental health practitioner who specializes in mind/body approaches — to help in your quest for better health and a longer life, take heed. Don't make that well-meaning person wheedle, cajole, and beg you to do something good for yourself. Remember "must syndrome"? That seems to include putting everyone else's needs first. Women *must* learn to recognize the signs that they need help managing stress or anger, or ending depression or anxiety.

Here are some concrete tips that you can implement today to help strengthen your emotional health:

Losing so many people in such a short time made me stop and wonder if I could do something to bring more meaning back into my life. Married to my high school sweetheart, beautiful little girls of my own, and a great job as a licensed court reporter — but still there was an emptiness in me. I decided to volunteer some of my time. Volunteering is tricky; the "who and how much" are very important decisions. In my fragile mental state, I made some unfortunate decisions.

My own personality — a dynamite work ethic combined with naiveté and a desire to excel at everything — made the uncomplicated task of volunteering turn into a full-time job that took over my life. Those were by far the hardest, most demanding, unrewarding, uncompensated years a person could have. At the end of that long stretch, working day and night helping others, I helped myself into sickness and a shattered heart.

Enter the liver disease that I told you about in Chapter 1.

The heart and liver rest inside the chest, as a size 6 shoe

- Understand what triggers a stress response for you. Either eliminate the trigger or find new ways to cope.
- Develop a daily relaxation practice: yoga, meditation, journal writing, biofeedback, guided imagery, walking, etc.
- Limit exposure to negative people and events.
- Develop an optimistic outlook. You don't need to be a Pollyanna, but when the odds are with you, you have every right — and deserve — to feel positive.
- Increase positive social support. Join a club, volunteer, get active in church, etc.
- Talk to a psychotherapist if you have stress, anxiety, depression, or excessive anger that doesn't resolve within a few weeks after your efforts to change.

Your physical health doesn't end at the invisible line that you've drawn between your body and your brain. Your physical health largely depends on your emotional well-being. If you have cardiac disease or wish to prevent it, all the fish oil and 30-minute walks you can possibly do may not be enough if you are unhappy. As a woman, you deserve a better quality of life. Change is always possible, and if you cannot do it alone, help from your physician or a health psychologist is always available.

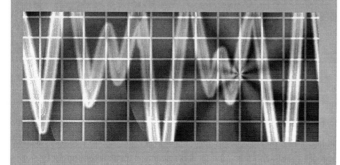

would fit in a box with a size 10 shoe: size 10 the liver, size 6 the heart. (Actually a person's heart is about the size of their fist.) During the months on Interferon, I would often lie in the fetal position and think about the pain my sickness brought. Liver disease is completely debilitating. Every single inch of your skin crawls and the nausea is relentless, which in turn causes weakness. The weakness is not relieved by sleep, because while you are trying to sleep the disease keeps you up with its unforgiving symptoms.

I could not turn off the switch in my mind that kept replaying, over and over again, the years I spent frantically trying to please others and to change the world for the better. The heartache I felt! I wish that I'd had the power to separate the emotion from the sickness so that I could see how bad I would feel physically — if emotionally I were not also so sick. I felt as if there were two separate people living inside my body. One Lois was sick with liver disease; the other Lois was sick from heartbreak.

When people say, "I have a broken heart," I see that literally as a broken heart that aches like a sore muscle. The heart is a muscle. As with any muscle that has been injured, bruised, cut, or torn, recovery can be slow. Time, therapy, and professional care are the usual recommendations.

If only we could apply a cast or a Band-Aid, others would see our broken heart. Be careful not to push us, we could say; we have a broken heart. We could have better seating, better parking, and perhaps people would ask us how our hearts became broken. We could share with them, and moan and groan together over the gory details of the break. Alas, our heart is hidden, and with this type of injury we're not supposed to act any differently on the job or among our peers. Sure, a heart can be healed with time, but *only* with time — and life is time.

I have learned — the hard way, of course — how depression and stress play a part in cardiovascular ills. In one article I read, "Taking Stress to Heart," Dr. Wei Jiang, an assistant professor of psychiatry and behavior at Duke University Medical Center in Durham, North Carolina, said that psychological factors can create "invisible damage," and that emotional distress appears to have a negative effect on the cardiovascular system. The lack of blood flow to the heart, a condition known as ischemia, can contribute to heart disease and other cardiac problems, she points out. In a worst-case scenario, the stress can lead to a heart attack.

Dr. David Sheps, associate chair of cardiovascular medicine at the University of Florida and editor-in-chief of the journal *Psychosomatic Medicine*, has studied the topic for more than 15 years. Although the mind-body link is complex, his research has consistently supported the notion that mental stress-induced ischemia can prove deadly — particularly among those already suffering from heart problems. While physical stress often produces symptoms, including chest pain, psychological factors can silently create damage.

Think about this: We make sure that our nails and our hair look terrific, and we buy all sorts of skin products. But our heart? Somehow we overlook the urgency of making our hearts a top-priority issue also. And, for the record, heart disease is not pretty.

Here's another issue that we often choose to ignore: On more than one occasion I allowed myself to be less of who I could be just to please others. Sure, I wanted to watch my diet, but because my boss might be a little overweight and I didn't want to hurt her feelings, I'd agree to join her at a fast food restaurant, and then get the combo meal rather than eat my healthy lunch from home. Who was I helping? I could have been a better example to my boss by declining the offer. Instead, I didn't want to offend, so I opted to be unhealthy, rather than do what I knew was best for myself.

I have these words from Nelson Mandela posted on my computer. Truly they are words around which we can build our lives:

> Our deepest fear is not that we are inadequate. Our deepest fear is that we are powerful beyond measure. It is our light, not our darkness, that frightens us. We ask ourselves, who am I to be brilliant, gorgeous, talented, and fabulous?
>
> Actually who are you not to be? You are a child of God. Your playing small doesn't serve the world. There's nothing enlightening about shrinking so other people won't feel insecure around you.
>
> We were born to manifest the Glory of God that is within us. It's not just in some; it's in all, everyone. And as we let our own light shine we unconsciously give other people permission to do the same. As we are liberated from our own fear, our presence automatically liberates others.
>
> — Nelson Mandela, 1994 Inaugural Speech

For too long, I had allowed myself to do the bidding of others — no matter how ill-advised it may have been — without a simple please or thank-you in return. No longer! Following my heart attack and subsequent diagnosis, I made up my mind that in the future I would hold to my purpose in life. I would not waste my future in toiling feverishly for people who cared nothing for others.

Please understand me: I didn't ask for my heart to ache for others. I didn't teach myself to cry at the slightest story of love, compassion, or renewed friendship. It's just the way I am; it's the way I've always lived my life. And now, my new mission: writing and speaking about women's heart disease, my own heart disease. My own heart.

Daily putting into practice what I teach others is an enormous test in itself. Yes, there's stress involved, and we know *that's* not a good thing. But sometimes, as I'm about to speak to a new group of women, I imagine my own coterie of supporters sitting in the back of the room. It gives me heart (if you'll excuse the expression).

There's my dad, and he looks great, though the rims of his glasses are larger than I'd remembered. And my grandmother, sitting next to him! No one has ever cooked any better than my grandmother; her stocky stature is a reminder of that. My dad's brothers are there, too, and they look so much like him, taller, but with that Stewart family face you'd know anywhere. My grandfather looks exactly like the pictures I've seen of him — so handsome, like the accountant in *Schindler's List*.

As I'm preparing to begin speaking, I see my father mouthing the words, "I'm very proud of you!" There's a goal I had always strived to accomplish. And having these dear departed members of my family in the room with me affirms for me that what I'm doing by sharing my story with women everywhere is changing lives that might have been stolen by heart disease, just as my dad's life was cut short.

Writing this chapter was so difficult! Many days I'd write only three or four sentences and need to take a nap. Allowing myself to travel back into my memories caused me to swim around deep waves of hurt longer than I anticipated. It showed me who I have been and unlocked some doors that had not only been shut, but also blocked by nearly impenetrable walls. Truly I hated to hear my cardiologist say to me that what I did in my twenties is why I have heart disease today.

But looking back at my life, perhaps he was right after all.

Chapter 4

Women's Heart 101

Now you've heard my story — well, an awful lot of it, anyway. You know about my battle with the elephant of heart disease, and about the characteristics of my family background that contributed to my susceptibility to heart disease. So enough about me already. Let's take a close look at what you need to know about your heart. This chapter could help you save your own life.

Remember: Heart disease is a *now* problem. Later might be too late.

Your heart beats an average of 70 beats per minute; in an hour that adds up to 4,200 beats. In 24 hours that's more than 100,000 beats. In a year your heart beats close to 37 million times. And by the time you're 50 years old, that's approximately 1,800,000,000 beats. All that time, your heart has been beating 24 hours a day, seven days a week.

An organ that works so unceasingly hard for you deserves the proper attention and care, right?

So what is heart disease really? It's when our heart doesn't get enough nutrient-rich blood. Heart disease can become chronic because often we don't know when trouble has been developing, often over many years. The condition known as atherosclerosis causes our arteries to harden as cholesterol, fat, and other substances build up in the artery walls; blockage can result in a heart attack. If not "fixed" by surgery or medical interventions (such as bypass, angioplasty, or medication), the condition will worsen, which can lead to disability or death. Heart disease *can* be prevented or controlled. Treatment includes lifestyle changes and, if needed, medication.

Now don't give up on me here. *Stay with me*! This is what we have to know. You might be tempted to think, "Oh, I already know this!" But please: Read this chapter as if it were a juicy, gossipy, personal story that someone has e-mailed to you by mistake.

Factors Within Your Control That Increase Women's Risk of Heart Disease

Listed below are actions that women can take that have the power to prevent or control heart disease.

Smoking. About 22.7 million women smoke. Women who smoke are six times more likely to have a heart attack than those who don't smoke. Luckily, you can reverse the damaging effects of smoking if you quit now.

High Blood Pressure or Hypertension. About 30% of women have hypertension (the condition's medical name). Uncontrolled high blood pressure can lead to heart failure, which affects about 2.5 million women. High blood pressure can often be hereditary, but it can be regulated with medication. You can help yourself by:

- following a healthy eating pattern;
- reducing salt and sodium in your diet;
- maintaining a healthy weight;
- being physically active; and
- limiting your intake of alcohol.

High blood pressure, or hypertension, is defined in an adult as a systolic pressure of 140 mm Hg or higher and/or a diastolic pressure of 90 mm Hg or higher. Blood pressure is measured in millimeters of mercury (mm Hg).

Blood Pressure (mm Hg)	Normal	Prehypertension	Hypertension
Systolic (top number)	less than 120	120-139	140 or higher
Diastolic (bottom number)	less than 80	80-89	90 or higher

High blood pressure can occur in children or adults. It's particularly prevalent in African-Americans, middle-aged and elderly people, obese people, and heavy drinkers. People with diabetes mellitus, gout, or kidney disease have hypertension more frequently. Of all those who have high blood pressure, 11% are not on medication, 25% are on medication but don't have their condition under control, and 34% are on adequate medication and have their hypertension under control.

The cause of 90–95% of the cases of high blood pressure isn't known; however, this disease is easily detected and usually controllable. High blood pressure directly increases the risk of coronary heart disease (which leads to heart attack) and stroke, especially when other risk factors are present. High blood pressure usually has no symptoms. It is truly a silent killer. But a simple, quick, painless test can detect it.

Diabetes. Diabetes is known to raise triglycerides and lower the amount of so-called "good cholesterol," or HDL. A low level of HDL has been shown to be the most powerful forecaster of heart disease. A high level of sugar in the blood also has a toxic effect on the walls of your arteries. Increased glucose, combined with cholesterol, increases the risk of developing atherosclerosis (also known as hardening of the arteries). This is a normal process of aging, but occurs at an accelerated rate in people with diabetes.

Ninety-five percent of the people I encountered at cardio rehab had diabetes as well as heart disease. So, women with diabetes, take care of yourself, the health of your heart is also at stake!

High Cholesterol. About 55 million women have high total cholesterol. What is cholesterol?

When I was first told I had plaque in my carotid artery, I had to ask the nurses what plaque was. Cholesterol is plaque; it's a waxy substance produced by the liver. It's also found in foods we eat that come from animals, such as meats, egg yolks, shellfish, and whole milk dairy products. When our bodies make too much cholesterol or too much is absorbed from the foods we eat, it's deposited in our arteries as plaque.

There are two kinds of cholesterol:

- "Bad" cholesterol, or LDL (low-density lipoproteins), clogs your arteries and puts you at risk for heart disease. LDL cholesterol is called bad because it's the type that gets stuck inside the walls of your blood vessels. And I used to think that LDL just stood for Lousy Cholesterol!
- "Good" cholesterol, or HDL (high-density lipoproteins), actually helps to remove bad cholesterol from your body. HDL lipoproteins are called good because they find and pick up stuck cholesterol, and return them to your liver.
- Triglycerides are a separate category. Triglycerides are particles made up of a small sugar-like molecule and three attached fatty acid molecules. They can be dangerous, too. Triglycerides are the chemical form in which most fat exists in food as well as in the body. Triglycerides in blood plasma are derived from fats eaten in foods or made in the body from other energy sources like carbohydrates. Calories ingested in a meal and not used immediately by your tissues are converted to triglycerides and transported to fat cells to be stored. Hormones regulate the release of triglycerides from fat tissue so they meet the body's needs for energy between meals.

Elevated levels of triglycerides have been linked to the occurrence of coronary artery disease in some people and may also be a consequence of other disease, such as untreated diabetes mellitus. Like cholesterol, increases in triglyceride levels can be detected by plasma measurements (after an overnight food and alcohol fast).

It's important to know, among other things, that simply taking some form of statin, or cholesterol-reducing medication, doesn't give us carte blanche to eat anything and everything we want. (As I had personally hoped it would!) We still have to watch what we eat, because non-nutritious delicacies filled with white flour and sugar could raise our triglyceride levels and cause heart disease just the same.

How Do You Know if Your Cholesterol Is High?

Many people simply do not know. High cholesterol is often referred to as a "silent disease." People with high cholesterol usually don't have any symptoms. That's why it's so important for adults to have their cholesterol screened at least every five years. Yearly, we women are supposed to see a gynecologist. Use that visit to have your cholesterol level checked, too; if it's high, insist on being referred to a cardiologist.

Be equipped. Know what your numbers mean and what they should be. New women's heart guidelines urge more aggressive treatment. The new guidelines issued by the American Heart Association (AHA) recommend treatment for women based on their levels of risk: high risk, intermediate risk, and lower risk. These guidelines call for women to have slightly higher levels of HDL, or "good" cholesterol, than men. They recommend a greater use of cholesterol-lowering medicines, especially for women at high risk for heart attacks even with normal cholesterol levels.

The optimal goal for total cholesterol is 200 milligrams per deciliter of blood (mg/dL), but the real bull's-eye target is your level of low-density lipoprotein (LDL) cholesterol, which nestles in artery walls and blocks blood flow. According to the

Healthy Goals for Women	
☐ Total Cholesterol	Less than 200 mg/dL
☐ LDL (bad) Cholesterol	*LDL cholesterol goals vary.
☐ HDL (good) Cholesterol	50 mg/dL or higher
☐ Triglycerides	Less than 150 mg/dL
☐ Blood Pressure	Less than 120/80 mmHg
☐ Fasting Glucose	Less than 110 mg/dL
☐ Body Mass Index (BMI)	Less than 25 Kg/m2
☐ Waist circumference	Less than 35 inches

*For people who don't have heart disease and one or no risk factors, the goal is less than 160 mg/dL.

Follow These Guidelines for a More Healthful Diet

Meats, Poultry, and Fish

Instead of:

High-fat meats
Fatback and bacon

Try:

Lean meats, poultry without skin, fish
Bean and grain dishes
Skinless chicken or turkey thighs

Cured Meats

Instead of:

Pork bacon
Pork sausage, ground beef, and pork

Try:

Turkey bacon, lean ham, Canadian
Ground skinless turkey breast

Dairy Products

Instead of:

Whole milk
Whole milk cheeses
Cream, evaporated milk
Sour cream

Try:

Skim (nonfat) or 1% milk
Low-fat or part skim milk cheeses
Evaporated skim milk
Low-fat yogurt

Fats, Spreads, and Dressings

Instead of:

Lard, butter, shortening
Regular mayonnaise,
regular salad dressing

Try:

Small amounts of vegetable oil
Mustard and nonfat or low-fat types of
salad dressing, yogurt, or mayonnaise

Here is a quick "sizing-up" of a serving:

One serving	Visual
½ cup dry cereal	Billiard ball
2 cups raw, leafy vegetables	2 baseballs
8 ounces yogurt	Tea cup
1 small apple or 1 medium orange	Tennis ball
½ baked potato	Computer mouse
½ bagel	Hockey puck
½ cup cooked pasta or rice	Ice cream scoop
½ cup sliced fruit	Light bulb
3 ounces chicken	Deck of cards
3 ounces fish	Checkbook
2 tablespoons raisins	Small egg
2 ounces hard cheese	Size C battery
1½ teaspoons peanut butter	Two dice
1 teaspoon butter or margarine	Tip of your thumb

Adult Treatment Panel III (ATPIII), a set of guidelines developed by the government, optimal LDL levels should be less than 100 milligrams per mg/dL, while levels of high-density lipoprotein (HDL) levels should be more than 50 mg/dL. Those with higher cardiovascular risk benefit by even lower LDL-C levels, below 70 mg/dL.

About 45% of women may need some form of statin, a family of cholesterol-lowering drugs.

Overweight/obesity. About 62% of U.S. women are overweight, including about 34% who are obese. We have been inundated with every diet on the market. We know what we should be doing for ourselves, and we know the many options that are available to us. Sometimes we just need a little trick to get started.

Here's my trick: for every 10 grams of fruit or cereal fiber you swallow daily, your risk of dying from heart disease falls by 27%. (I found this tidbit in a review of 10 studies from the Archives of Internal Medicine.) Shoot for a total of 25-30 grams of fiber from all sources each day. Do this gradually. I became so excited with the facts that I added the 30 grams of fiber to my diet instantly, and my family moved out of the house! Just kidding. But eat fiber — lots of fiber!

It's amazing: Year after year, heart disease remains the number-one killer of American men and women. Nearly 62 million Americans of all ages have cardiovascular diseases, according to the American Heart Association. And yet *a healthful low-fat eating plan, combined with regular physical activity, is the key to heart health*. Eat foods low in saturated fat and cholesterol.

For lunch I'm having a hockey puck with two dice, a side of teacup, and a tennis ball for dessert.

Seriously, after every seminar I'm asked what I eat, how I eat, and how my eating habits have changed since being diagnosed with heart disease. The DASH (Dietary Approaches to Stop Hypertension) eating plan, from which I borrowed the guidelines above, was the diet explained to all of us who were part of the 3:30 Monday-Friday Cardio Rehabilitation Group. If you want to learn more about the DASH eating plan, type DASH Diet into any search engine, or use this handy link: www.health.gov/ dietaryguidelines/dga2005/document/html/appendixA.htm

I learned a lot about portion size, for example, by studying the DASH diet. Here's a sample of what I eat on a daily basis:

Breakfast: Yogurt with flaxseed, and whole wheat English muffin or seven-grain wheat bread with light heart-healthy margarine, coffee.

Lunch: I like sandwiches, and I use whole wheat pita bread, with fat-free lunch meat, tomatoes, lettuce, and cucumbers.

Dinner: Vegetables, fish, chicken, brown rice, and cut-up fruit.

On the first radio show we did together, Dr. Warren Johnston shared that a person can run five miles and go home and eat a candy bar — and the exercise really was just for that candy bar. Common sense is the best diet. We all know more than we will ever do. My personal downfall is chips and salsa. I buy soy chips and, except for the salt content, I don't feel too guilty while indulging. There you have it: nothing spectacular, all easy to find, especially if you have a ranch market near by.

The new food chart is available from the U.S. Department of Agriculture. (See www.mypyramid.gov/index.html) Enter your age, sex, and level of physical activity. Based on that information, the site provides a nutrition plan, based on 12 different amounts of total daily calories. The calorie amounts range from 1,000 to 3,200.

I'll confess that sticking to a proper diet has been a huge challenge for me, and has caused me much confusion and depression. However, having passed the third anniversary of the discovery of abundant plaque in my arteries, I'm getting the hang of it. When you think about it (and I do), all of us really do have enough information thrown at us to truly understand what we should and should not eat. Although, if that's truly the case, then why does the food court at the mall have absolutely nothing on anyone's recommended list?

Here's an important note: Let's not forget about the interaction (maybe especially for women) between food and stress. Confession time: On a good day (okay, most days now), my daily eating habits are aligned perfectly with what I described to you above. Turn those recommendations upside down, however, and you have Lois under stress. I refer to it as "power eating" — eating as quickly and as much as possible. The longer I hang over the sink with that brownie in my mouth, the longer it will be before I have to deal with whatever is stressing me out. Tell me you haven't felt just that way sometimes. Be honest! But I am *not* advocating power eating. I'm simply reminding you that the connection between stress and eating is yet another manifestation of the powerful connections between mind and body.

And since we're improving our eating habits, here's something else you can do. After the age of 2, our children need to be taught about eating heart-healthy foods. Why? Because studies suggest more than one in three kids could have abnormal blood fats that begin damaging their little arteries early in life. Many pediatricians now recommend that children age 2 and older who are overweight and have a family history of high cholesterol, high blood pressure, diabetes, early heart attack, or stroke should be tested for these risk factors.

A sidelight here, in line with the theme of this book: I've seen a great ad that shows a cute little boy; the voiceover says, "At 4 he troubles your heart" and then "At 40 his heart might trouble him." In light of all we know, it would be appropriate to also show a little girl.

Physical Inactivity. Unfortunately, more women than men are physically inactive. About 27% of women engage in no leisure-time physical activity, and about 60% do not meet the recommended exercise level of at least 30 minutes a day of such moderately intense activity as brisk walking. While it's also true heart disease is "ageless," no matter what a woman's age, she needs to take action to protect her heart health.

> Obviously, volatile emotions such as anger and hostility are bad for your heart's health. But studies have also shown that some of the quieter emotions can be just as toxic and damaging.

As women we simply do not make our health a top priority. It's not deliberate. We really mean to, but there is only so much we can fit into our calendar. We feel too busy to make changes in our lives. It's easy to say that we need to add 30 minutes of exercise most days of the week, but did anyone say which part of the day? Getting up earlier and leaving the house doesn't always work, because many of us have children and husbands who need our help in the mornings. And if I try to work out in the morning, my hair looks lousy afterwards. So, if I go to the gym before work, I also have to build in enough time to shower and blow-dry my hair. I have thought of shaving it, but I'm not ready for that look. Neither is my husband. It's no wonder that we see all these "30-Minute Workout" gyms popping up all over the place.

We have all read that exercise releases endorphins into our bloodstream, which actually reduce stress and help us relax. Exercise helps to bring our cholesterol down. If only exercise could be in pill form! And if you're already tired — if you're a recovering heart patient, for example, and you wake up tired — it's pretty darned hard to motivate yourself for a brisk workout. You know I'm right! Well, forgive me, I don't mean to give you any more excuses to avoid doing what you know you should do. And we know what we should do: Use the stairs instead of the elevator. Park a little farther away and walk instead of getting all stressed out trying to find a close parking space. Yeah, we've heard it. Now let's do it. It's simple.

Stress/Depression Link. There is a link between heart disease and depression. Depressed post-menopausal women have a 50% greater risk of developing or dying from heart disease than those who are not depressed, raising the possibility that treating the mind could help the body fight cardiovascular ills. This finding came from a four-year government study of 100,000 women across the United States. What is most striking is that depression was found to be an independent risk factor for subsequent cardio-vascular death.

Obviously, volatile emotions such as anger and hostility are bad for your heart's health. But studies have also shown that some of the quieter emotions can be just as toxic and damaging. Dr. Dean Ornish said, "Study after study has shown that people who feel lonely, depressed, and isolated are many times more likely to get sick and die prematurely, not only of heart disease but from virtually all causes, than those who have a sense of connection, love, and community."

In cases of depression, women outnumber men 2-1. Women seem to adopt the "tend and befriend" attitude; they internalize their anger and disappointment instead of expressing these emotions, and they become nicer and more nurturing. Quiet people who hold everything in can experience a great increase in stress reactions. Women commonly put themselves last on the list and feel too pressed for time to exercise or give themselves down time. (Research in this area was conducted by researchers at Johns Hopkins University and cited in the *New England Journal of Medicine*.)

Factors Beyond Your Control That Increase Women's Risk of Heart Disease

- Age: 55 or older. Risk rises between the ages of 40 and 60.
- Estrogen Level: A woman's estrogen level drops during menopause.
- Heredity: A family history of early heart disease increases your chance of having it too.

My own two cents here: we already read of the link between stress and depression, but these factors we can't change are *most* depressing. Earlier I wrote about my own family history of heart disease. Unbelievable as it may seem, however, at *no* time in my life had any doctor — even my favorite ones — talked to me with concern about my family history, cholesterol levels, the implications of a hyster-ectomy, or my lifestyle as a means of preventing heart disease. Did the entire medi-cal profession during those years believe heart disease was a man's disease? Maybe so.

Listed below are warning signs of impending heart attack. Women often don't recognize that they're having a heart attack and may ignore the signs.

Experts say to call 9-1-1 if you have one or more of these symptoms:

- Chest pain or discomfort. Most heart attacks start slowly, with mild pain or discomfort, usually in the center of the chest. It can feel like uncomfortable pressure, squeezing, fullness, or pain.
- Discomfort in the stomach, jaw, neck, or back. Women frequently feel this type of pain, either in addition to or without the chest pain. From my own experience, and that of many other women, this occurs commonly as upper back pain between the shoulder blades. Don't wait, as I did. Call 9-1-1.
- Shortness of breath
- Cold sweat
- Nausea or feelings of indigestion. Here's a tricky situation, because I was sent home from the hospital with the diagnosis of indigestion. Remember: most of us have experienced indigestion, so this isn't the typical "I'll pop a few antacids" indigestion. This is a burning sensation where your intuition tells you something much more is going on. Again, don't be embarrassed if it is indigestion. It could be anxiety, as well.
- Lightheadedness accompanying any of these symptoms. (I knew I could not drive myself to the emergency room. I was lightheaded, extremely anxious, and had enough sense to ask my daughter to drive me.)

Surviving a Heart Attack

How do you survive a heart attack? Fast action is your best weapon. Clot-busting drugs and other artery-opening treatments can stop a heart attack in its tracks. They can prevent or limit damage to the heart, but they need to be given immediately after symptoms begin. The sooner such treatments are administered, the more good they will do, and the greater your chances for survival and full recovery. To be most effective, these treatments need to be given within *one hour* of the start of heart attack symptoms.

Uncertainty is normal. Expectations often don't match reality when it comes to heart attacks. People expect a heart attack to happen as it does in the movies, where someone clutches his or her chest in pain and falls over. Because of this expectation, people often are not sure if they're having a heart attack. As a result, there's often a tendency to take a wait-and-see approach instead of seeking care immediately. Believe it or not, this happens even to people who have already had a heart attack! They may not recognize the symptoms because their next heart attack can have entirely different symptoms. Delay can be deadly. Most persons having a heart attack wait too long to seek medical help, and that can be a fatal mistake. *Patient delay — not transport or hospital delay — is the biggest cause of people* not *receiving rapid care for heart attacks.*

Women do not understand the symptoms of a heart attack and often think that what they are feeling is due to something else. They are afraid or unwilling to admit that their symptoms could be serious. They're embarrassed about "causing a scene" or going to the hospital and finding out it's a false alarm. As a result, most heart attack victims wait two hours or more after their symptoms begin before they seek medical help. This delay can result in death or permanent heart damage. This damage can reduce your ability to do everyday activities. Please understand the importance of getting to the hospital right away!

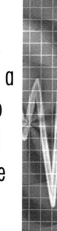

Delay can be deadly. Most persons having a heart attack wait too long to seek medical help, and that can be a fatal mistake.

The first step to take when a heart attack happens is easy: *Call 9-1-1*! Call whether or not you're sure you're having a heart attack. Anyone showing heart attack warning signs needs to receive medical treatment right away.

Don't wait more than a few minutes — five minutes at most — to call 9-1-1. Calling 9-1-1 for an ambulance is the best way to get to the hospital. Emergency medical personnel (also called EMS, for emergency medical services) can begin treatment even before arrival at the hospital.

The heart may stop beating during a heart attack. This is called Sudden Cardiac Arrest, and it accounts for more than 25% of the 500,000 deaths annually from women's heart disease. Emergency personnel have the equipment needed to start the heart beating again. Heart attack patients who arrive by ambulance tend to receive faster treatment on their arrival at the hospital.

Calling 9-1-1 is like bringing a hospital emergency department to your door. Emergency medical personnel can take vital signs, determine your medical condition, and if needed give added medical care. In many places, emergency medical personnel are linked to hospitals and doctors, so they can relay your vital signs and EKG results to the emergency department before you arrive. This way, you receive immediate continued treatment by emergency department personnel once you reach the hospital. If for some reason, you are having heart attack symptoms and cannot call 9-1-1, have someone immediately drive you to the hospital. Never drive yourself to the hospital, unless you absolutely have no other choice.

What to Do if You Are Alone and Having a Heart Attack

The best strategy is to be aware of the early warning signs for heart attack and cardiac arrest and respond to them by calling 9-1-1. If you're driving alone and you start having severe chest pain or discomfort that begins to spread into your arm and up into your jaw, pull over and flag down another motorist for help, or phone 9-1-1 on a cellular telephone.

(Incidentally, you may have seen the Internet instructions on surviving a heart attack if you are alone. These instructions — involving repeated, vigorous coughing — are a hoax, however, and are not endorsed by the American Heart Association or the Red Cross.) This coughing technique to maintain blood flow during brief arrhythmias has been used under controlled conditions in the hospital, particularly during cardiac catheterization. In such cases the patient's EKG is monitored continuously, and a physician is present. During cardiac catheterization, patients may develop sudden arrhythmias. If a life-threatening arrhythmia is detected within the first 10 to 15 seconds and before the patient loses consciousness, a physician or nurse may tell the patient to cough. Repeated, forceful coughing can help the person stay conscious until the arrhythmia disappears or is treated. Therefore, the usefulness of "cough CPR" is generally limited to monitored patients with a witnessed arrest in a hospital setting.

The Best Advice: Plan Ahead!

1. Learn the heart attack warning signs.

2. Think through what you would do if you had heart attack symptoms. Decide what you would do if it happened while you were at home, in the middle of the night, at work, or at any other place or in any other situation that might need advance planning.

3. Decide who would care for any dependents in an emergency. Emergency medical personnel will generally contact a friend or relative (or the police department, if necessary) to make emergency arrangements for your dependents.

4. Talk with your family and friends about the heart attack warning signs and the importance of acting fast by calling 9-1-1 after a few minutes (five minutes at the most), if those signs persist. Explain the benefits of calling 9-1-1, instead of getting to the hospital by car.

5. Gather important information to take with you to the hospital. You can do this by preparing a heart attack survival plan. Here are some suggestions. Print them out and keep copies in handy places, such as your wallet or purse.

- A list of the medicines you are taking
- A list of the medicines you're allergic to
- Your doctor's phone number during office hours
- The first person to contact if you go to the hospital: name, phone number at work, home, and mobile phone

Again, these things should be done when you're feeling healthy and well. You won't have time to prepare lists of medications and phone numbers if you are in the middle of a heart attack.

Here is a mind-boggling idea. Have a heart-to-heart talk with your doctor. The following is a great checklist; take it with you to your doctor appointment, or write your own questions.

- What is my risk for heart disease?
- What is my blood pressure? What does it mean for me, and what do I need to do about it?
- What are my cholesterol numbers? (These include total cholesterol, LDL, HDL, and triglycerides, a type of fat found in the blood and food.) What do they mean for me and what do I need to do about them?
- What is "body mass index" and waist measurement? Do they indicate that I need to lose weight for my health?
- What is my blood sugar level, and does it mean I'm at risk for diabetes? If so, what do I need to do about it?
- What other screening tests for heart disease do I need?
- Why do I have dark hairs growing out of my chin? (Just kidding — seeing if you're paying attention!)
- What can you do to help me quit smoking?
- How much physical activity do I need to help protect my heart?
- What is a heart-healthy eating plan for me?
- How can I tell if I may be having a heart attack? If I think I'm having one, what should I do?

Use these questions. Have them ready before you visit your doctor. Tell your doctor your lifestyle behaviors such as smoking or being physically inactive. Be honest with him; he won't tell anyone. If every Sunday afternoon after church you go behind the garage when everyone thinks you're going upstairs for a nap and smoke two packs of cigarettes, tell him. Also, tell your doctor any symptoms you feel. Don't be embarrassed. Better embarrassed and wrong than *dead* wrong. My head has never tingled again in that spot and made me sneeze. Never. Therefore, opening whatever artery they opened up in the highway of arteries leading to or away from my heart somehow put an end to my head tingling.

Laughter

Have you laughed at all while reading this book? How about laughing while watching a great TV show? Can you even remember the last time you laughed? Catherine Kalamis, in "Laugh Your Way to Health" (*Choice* magazine, March 2001), said that a 10-minute bout of laughing can have the following effects:

- As the person laughs, carbon dioxide is driven out of the body and replaced by oxygen-rich air, providing physical and mental freshness.
- Laughing can produce anti-inflammatory agents that can aid back pain or arthritis.
- Laughing encourages muscles to relax and exercises muscles all over the body, from the scalp to the legs.
- Laughing reduces levels of cortisol, the stress hormone.
- It is also thought that laughter may possibly aid immune system responses, (though the evidence for that is primarily anecdotal).
- Laughing exercises facial muscles to prevent sagging.
- Laughing boosts the production of "feel-good" endorphin hormones.

A study performed at the University of Maryland noted that laughter seems to cause the tissue that forms the inner lining of blood vessels to relax or expand, increasing blood flow. Mental stress, on the other hand, causes the opposite effect: making vessels constrict, and thus reducing blood flow. That finding confirms earlier studies that suggest a link between emotional stress and the narrowing of these linings, called the endothelium.

The endothelium is the layer of thin, flat cells that lines the interior surface of blood vessels. Endothelial cells line the entire circulatory system, from the heart to the smallest capillary. In small blood vessels and capillaries, endothelial cells are often the only type of cell present. Endothelial cells are involved in many aspects of vascular biology, including:

- Vasoconstriction and vasodilation, and hence the control of blood pressure
- Blood clotting (thrombosis and fibrinolysis)
- Atherosclerosis

- Formation of new blood vessels (angiogenesis)
- Inflammation and swelling (edema)

So: Stress is bad. Laughing is good. We all have stress, so before you put this book down and curl up in the fetal position, I have great news. Really.

Chocolate (Really!)

Research suggests that CHOCOLATE (yes, it deserves to be capitalized) meets a variety of needs. I know, I know, there's that whole thing about chocolate and the libido, but this is a serious book! I'm writing about the chocolate and your heart. Chocolate seems to straddle the line between a food and a beneficial medicine. Even the conventional wisdom that chocolate is related to acne has been challenged. Its chemical properties are complicated, as is the choice on which kind of chocolate to eat or where to purchase it. (That's so me writing there.)

Chocolate contains more than 300 substances, including caffeine in small quantities, and theobromine, a weaker stimulant. Some contend that these two chemicals form the basis of the much-touted chocolate high, postulating that they increase activity of key neurotransmitters. The stimulant phenylethylamine, which is related chemically to amphetamines, is also in chocolate.

This particular section on chocolate and its benefits have opened up a river of deep, dark (sometimes light) experiences. Make no mistake, with this research I have chomped into I find myself a little kinder while enjoying this derivative from the ancient Maya and Aztec civilizations.

Pets

Pets provide unconditional love and companionship for people of all ages — a fact that any pet owner can confirm. But scientific research also suggests pets help people control blood pressure and manage stress. Researchers have taken an interest in pets because controlling stress and blood pressure are vital keys to reducing the risk of heart disease, heart attack, and stroke. A 2000 study, for instance, found that dogs help relieve cardiovascular stress in people who have had difficulty controlling their stress.

The study was just one of a series that demonstrated the positive health benefits of pet ownership. Dr. Karen Allen has led a team of researchers from the State University of New York (SUNY) at Buffalo in a series of pet-related studies that began more than a decade ago. Their results have repeatedly demonstrated that people show a reduced stress response (i.e., less of a rise in blood pressure or heart rate) if their pet happens to be nearby. Pets comfort us when we face life's many challenges.

The SUNY-Buffalo research team has also studied the effects of owning a pet on a group of hypertensive people who were caring for their brain-injured spouses. Half of the caregivers adopted a dog for six months. At the end of those six months, the new pet owners were reacting to stress better than they had before, and better than the caregivers who did not have a pet. The other half of the caregivers then adopted a dog. After another six months, all of the caregivers were reacting better to stress.

Research has found that health benefits are not limited to dogs or (by extension) cats. A study found that watching brightly colored fish swim back and forth in an aquarium helped calm people prone to disruptive behavior, such as children with attention deficit/hyperactivity disorder.

Nursing homes in both the United States and Europe have documented the helpful effects of bringing in pets to visit the residents, and many people have benefited from therapeutic programs that allow them to interact with horses, dolphins, and other animals.

Exactly why pets can have a positive physiological effect is not clear, but experts have a number of theories. Research in general has shown that people tend to be healthier when they have a companion. In addition, studies have shown that people enjoyed more social interaction if they were accompanied by a dog. It may also be that people have an easier time reaching out to a pet than to a person! Pets bridge all communication gaps.

At the beginning of my New Life Adjustments, I tried to play my part by finding every fat-free, cholesterol-free, sugar-free food I could and eating them all in one day. I tried hard to be the perfect patient. Just when I thought I had made some strides with boundaries, however, I realized that my many years *without* boundaries had caught up with me and played a part in my heart disease! I woke up some mornings so depressed that I deliberately chose not to work out, but to have a hamburger and fries instead. Not often, but it happened. A death wish? No, it was a matter of bumping up against a new (and very unpleasant) reality — the reality of being told what I am not allowed to eat for the rest of my life and then sometimes rebelling at the drive-through window. I used to look at people who I knew had health problems as they gobbled down their cake and soda at a party and think, not *me*. Never would *I* take my health for granted. Hmm. . .

Who was I kidding? Isn't putting work or other people ahead of yourself or your family — as I allowed myself to do — just as bad as eating fries and a hamburger for breakfast? Saying "yes" when your mind and your body are screaming "no" is equally as detrimental to your health as having too much alcohol. Many things we think, do, and experience are not healthy.

I'm coming to grips these days with the reality that only one person can change this: me. And my aim in this chapter has been to pass along to you the best of what we know about diet, exercise, dealing with heart attacks and their symptoms, and wellness research. In the next chapter we'll talk about tests and treatments — but from the patient's point of view.

The Mind-Body Feedback Loop: An Endocrinologist's Perspective of Stress and Cardiometabolic Disease

Jannet Huang, MD, FRCPC, FACE

Cardiovascular disease (heart attack, stroke, etc.) continues to be on the rise as the leading cause of death in the United States, as well as the cause of devastating decline in women's quality of life (a fact that is, unfortunately, seldom acknowledged). This is true despite the increasing number of medications being used to treat blood pressure and cholesterol — medications that have actually led to a decrease in mortality in men from coronary heart disease.

Why have women not been blessed with the same downward trend? There are many explanations, including such issues as inadequate awareness on the part of both women and their physicians, the often different and more subtle symptoms among women, and the fact that women are more susceptible to non-classical risk factors that include psycho-social stressors.

I am sure that the story of Lois Trader, our lady in the red dress, is striking a chord in many readers. Her powerful story is by no means unique, but she has the vision and courage to speak up and share her life so that other women can be more aware and therefore be more proactive about their cardiovascular health.

Endocrinologists are at the forefront of research into the hormonal mechanisms of the profound effects of stress on our bodies. In this short addition to Lois' book, I would like to share some recent research findings, which I hope may motivate you to raise yourselves up in your priority list, to balance and center your lifestyle, and to avoid the adverse cardiovascular outcomes that may be just lurking around the corner.

I decided to use "The Mind-Body Feedback Loop" as my title because a feedback loop is the way in which most of our endocrine system functions. For example, the thyroid hormones (produced by the thyroid gland) are monitored by the pituitary, the master gland of the endocrine system. When thyroid levels are too low, this signals the pituitary gland, which in turn stimulates the thyroid gland to work harder and rev up its production process. This feedback mechanism allows the hormone-producing glands and the pituitary to communicate constantly, thereby keeping us in homeostasis — a state of balance. I believe that the mind and the body also operate with a feedback loop that operates constantly to keep us in balance. Unfortunately, a lot of us ignore our body's signals to our mind, pushing on and on even when we are exhausted and spent.

Maybe you yourself have made of these comments to yourself or to others:

- "I'm so tired, my fatigue is deep in my bones!"
- "I can't get rid of this weight I gained in my abdomen despite improving my diet and exercise habits! Of course, I don't have much time to exercise, and I'm usually too tired anyway. I'm so discouraged."
- "There must be something wrong physically in my body!"

Today's environment poses a lot of challenges to our bodies. People's lifestyles have changed so rapidly in the last century that our genes cannot possibly evolve fast enough to adapt. Our ancestors evolved in an environment of unpredictable food supply; genetic traits that favored the storage of fat were positively selected in the evolutionary process.

However, genetic traits that enhanced the chances of survival in prehistoric times are now detrimental in our times of overabundance. The advent of processed foods and the abundance of nutritionally deprived but calorically-dense portions, along with our diminished levels of physical activity, have created obesity and other lifestyle diseases such as heart disease, diabetes, and certain cancers. Our ancestors used to hunt and forage for food, and their diet consisted of mainly fruits and high-fiber vegetation as well as some lean protein. The meats they ate were higher-quality protein with less fat, since the wild animals they hunted ran from predators and were therefore much leaner! Our meat sources today are animals that are overfed and sedentary, so protein and fat are almost always intermingled. And let's not ignore the ballooning of portion sizes over the last 50 years. A Classic Coke in an eight-ounce glass bottle was 100 kilo-calories (kcal), whereas today an "extreme gulp" 52-ounce soft drink delivers a whopping 630 kcal! An old-time hamburger was 280 kcal; today's "double Whopper with cheese" packs in 1,120 kcal!

One of the common denominators of cardiometabolic risk is abdominal weight gain — an increase in visceral fat, also known as "belly fat." Increased caloric intake and decreased physical activity are not the only contributing factors, however. Stress and sleep deprivation are also major players. Visceral fat is the "bad fat" that produces inflammatory chemicals and releases more free fatty acids to the liver. This increase in visceral fat is a root cause of insulin resistance and type 2 diabetes, which leads to increased cardiovascular risk, which is also raised further by psychosocial stress.

Some scientists believe that sleep loss is a major contributing factor to our twin epidemics of obesity and diabetes. In the last 40 years, the percentage of Americans who report sleeping less than seven hours a night has increased from 16% to 37%. Normally, the body's cortisol level drops significantly after habitual bedtime, but the cortisol level of sleep-restricted people does not display the normal nocturnal drop. The resultant chronically elevated evening cortisol levels increase our risk of obesity and diabetes.

Moreover, appetite-controlling hormones are affected by the duration of sleep. In a state of sleep deprivation, the increase in hunger is out of proportion to the caloric demand of staying awake. Leptin is a hormone secreted by fat cells to signal satiety, or fullness, to the brain; its levels are reduced even by short-term sleep restriction. There is an associated increase in ghrelin, a hormone signaling hunger secreted by the stomach.

Changes in these appetite-regulating hormones were seen in normal subjects after as little as two nights of sleep restriction to four hours per night. In a study of healthy subjects, even after just six days of sleep restriction (four hours of sleep per night), there is a notable increase in blood sugar levels after breakfast. This study result supports the hypothesis that chronic sleep deprivation increases insulin resistance and type 2 diabetes.

The intimate link between insulin resistance/diabetes and cardiovascular disease is being confirmed repeatedly by research. A recent study showed that among patients with no prior diagnosis of diabetes who are admitted to the coronary care unit with their first heart attack, a glucose tolerance test (a rigorous, sensitive test for the presence of diabetes) shows that 31% are actually diabetic. Another 35% have impaired glucose tolerance ("pre-diabetes"), and only 34% are truly non-diabetic!

A growing body of research is confirming the profound effect of psychosocial stress on cardiovascular risk. The well-known INTERHEART study published in 2004 showed the likelihood of having a heart attack is increased by 42.3 times when a person has all four "traditional" heart risk factors (smoking, diabetes, hypertension, and hyperlipidemia). Here's an additional finding of this same study that is not so well-known: The likelihood of a heart attack is increased to 182.9 times if psychological stress is present in addition to the four traditional risk factors! In patients with acute cardiac illness, major depression is associated with a fourfold increase in mortality following a myocardial infarction. Anxiety is associated with a threefold higher risk of mortality following myocardial infarction, a twofold increase in risk of re-infarction over five years, and a sixfold higher risk of sudden cardiac death.

There is good news, however. There is now ample evidence that mind-body medicine strategies are effective in reducing cardiovascular risk. In order to prevent diabetes and cardiovascular disease, an integrative strategy is imperative. We must better understand our risk factors, both traditional and non-classical. We must allow the time and energy for self-care, with a healthy, balanced, sustainable lifestyle as the foundation. A diet that is high in fiber and rich in omega 3 fatty acids, plus antioxidants from fruits and vegetables, is a good start. Regular exercise is not only good for our cardiovascular health but also for our mental health. Exercise even reduces the likelihood of menopausal symptoms. What could be better than that? Stress reduction and improving sleep quality is paramount to our overall health. Evidence-based use of vitamin supplements and judicious use of pharmaceutical agents complement the program for diabetes and cardiovascular disease prevention.

I invite you to contemplate the meaning of "optimal health" — a state of balance and well-being that encompasses all layers of a human being: physical, mental, emotional, sexual, and spiritual. Don't wait! You too can get the tools you need to attain the state of optimal health.

Jannet Huang, MD, FRCPC, FACE, Endocrinology & Metabolism
Medical Director, The Center for Optimal Health
6825 Quail Hill Parkway, Irvine, CA 92603

Chapter 5

I've Had All These Tests Twice

Okay, now you've read through "Women's Heart 101." Maybe you knew a lot of what was in the previous chapter already. Or maybe I succeeded in raising your consciousness, as mine was raised (though less forcibly, I hope). Now you know all the useful information we've been told again and again, but have always managed to avoid dealing with. So you have another chance, just as I did, to make heart-saving knowledge a vital part of your everyday life.

Chapter 4 was aimed at helping you save your own life. This chapter is different. Picture me writing it while wearing my "Survivor" T-shirt — the one that always makes people ask if I mean the TV show. No, I mean that I've been through all the tests I describe in this chapter more than once. Believe me, I know my way around hospitals better than anyone would want to. So my aim in this chapter is to share with you some hard-earned information that may make your life easier and less anxious.

And here's an added bonus: My friend and colleague Dr. Warren Johnston — the cardiologist who wrote the Afterword you'll find at the end of this book — has provided his input to this chapter as well. He read through it meticulously and gave it his stamp of approval. You'll also find a thoughtful note from him to you, the reader, in this chapter.

Here's the role I'd like to play for you in this chapter. You know how, when you visit your neighborhood drugstore with a new prescription, the pharmacist asks if you have any questions? I want to be like that pharmacist, someone who can help you as you struggle to understand confusing (and sometimes conflicting) information, someone you have known and trusted for years. My purpose is to help you find your way down the road to knowing your own heart health — and to using your own smarts and power.

Truthfully, there are only so many tests that can possibly be prescribed for you, and

I've had all of them — every single procedure, blood test, and stress-related treadmill trip that you'll be likely to face. So think of me as your guide through the bewildering labyrinth of hospital corridors, and hospital procedures. Ladies, talking to me is like talking to your sister who had three children before you had your first baby. It's comforting to hear from someone who has actually been through it.

Now then, let's get going.

A Word to the Reader

As I read along with you, I feel the need to stop and applaud Lois Trader on her uncanny ability to discuss difficult and confusing medical terminology — not to mention diagnostic testing and treatment options — and make them simple and easy to understand.

This is truly a gift.

Like you, I enjoy reading Lois' opinions and laughing at her often humorous insights. I would be remiss, however, if I did not point out that modern-day medicine can indeed be complicated and confusing. Like most things in life, medical opinion is often controversial. It has been said that if you ask five cardiologists for an opinion you will get 10 opinions! While debate and disagreement can be healthy, often patients are left feeling bewildered.

It is important to remember, as Lois points out repeatedly, that *you* are your own best advocate. While your doctor remains your best resource to negotiate the complex medical system, if you feel that your questions are not being addressed to your satisfaction, by all means seek a second opinion. No doctor worth his (or her) salt would ever take offense at that!

So continue reading and learning from Lois and her life-changing experiences, and remember: *Make Yourself Your Best Cause!*

Yours in health,
Warren D. Johnston, MD, FACC, FACP

You are experiencing chest pain, shortness of breath, rapid pounding heartbeats, sweating, and a feeling of impending doom. You're a mess. You've tried to reason with yourself that you're only having, say, a panic attack — not a heart attack. After all, panic attacks are certainly common; many of us have experienced them at one time or another. You've read a few articles and talked with your friends. The body reacts to anxiety by producing stress hormones, and it's these stress hormones that are causing your symptoms, right?

But your chest continues to burn; dizziness, weakness, nausea, and severe indigestion (along with a heightened sense of anxiety) are flooding over you. Are you having a panic attack or a heart attack? Both can display similar symptoms, and panic attacks are nothing to scoff at. But symptoms that last for more than two or three minutes, or pain that leaves and then returns, could signal a heart attack. Only by having testing can a correct diagnosis be made.

You decide to go see your doctor — or maybe even go to the emergency room — because you can't talk yourself into believing you're having a panic attack. Good for you!

The **physical examination** is always the first stop on your journey to heart health. That walk down the hallway to the patient room never changes, does it? And somehow it's always necessary to step on that blasted scale — no matter how we're dressed or what time of day it is. (No doubt you've observed throughout this book my aversion to scales of all kinds.)

As a long-time patient I've learned some tricks, however. I try to make all my appointments early. I wear lightweight clothes and flip-flops, even if it's cold outside, in an attempt to reduce the dreaded scale shock. (Of course, I live in California.) Actually, I do know why they have to take your weight initially. It's because your body-mass index (BMI) is an important heart risk factor. Once we have that established, however, what woman wants to weigh herself continually?

Waiting, waiting in my puke-green gown open at the back. Hold on, since it's a checkup for my heart, should the opening be in the front instead? I'll be embarrassed if I put it on wrong. For the record, you won't find this checkup to be much different from any other checkup — blood pressure, pulse, listening to your heart with a stethoscope, questions about medications. Pretty much the usual drill.

Oh, and a **blood test** is prescribed. This test requires a 12-hour fasting period — no eating at all — before they draw your blood. I hate fasting, for any purpose! I look up the type of blood test that's on my prescription. Advanced lipid testing. Not everyone needs advanced lipid testing — I'm having this blood test after my diagnosis of heart disease. The advanced lipid testing is simply the designation for the in-depth process that directly measures the amount of lipids in your body. In the normal range, lipids are necessary for good health. But when lipids are out of the normal range, they may represent a risk factor associated with heart disease. If your lipids are out of normal range, you (and your doctor) have several options, including diet, exercise, and drug therapy that will help return them to normal and maintain the health of your heart and body.

Either way, though, your initial blood test will be a fasting blood test for blood count, basic blood profile that addresses kidney and liver function, blood sugar, albumin, and the electrolytes such as sodium, potassium, and calcium. The **full lipid profile** I mentioned immediately above really should be done, so be sure to ask if it has been ordered, since who can ever read the scribbles on a prescription form?

In addition, the advanced lipid testing measures total cholesterol, HDL and LDL cholesterol, and triglyceride levels; hs-CRP and Homocysteine are also ordered because they may show abnormalities that are predictive of heart disease. I advise you to ask that your thyroid function, called **TSH (thyroid-stimulating hormone)** be checked as well. An underactive thyroid can sometimes be associated with high cholesterol levels.

In addition, I've had an episode where my thyroid became hyper — overactive rather than underactive (called hyperthyroidism). It scared me because the symptoms of hyperthyroidism seemed to mimic the symptoms of a heart attack. My heart was having unusual palpitations, I had cold sweats, and I felt really lousy. So you might consider asking to have that TSH blood test; since they already have that needle in your arm, what's another tube of blood? That's how I look at it.

What I don't like about full lipid profiles is that usually they can't be performed in your familiar local doctor's office. Because it's a complicated blood test, in my area, for instance, there are only two places to choose from. Both are overcrowded, and being there makes me feel like I'm sicker than I am. I've learned to leave an hour before these labs are open, bring a book or newspaper, and just sit outside and relax, trying to be one of the first patients. You can't eat or drink coffee anyway, so why not get out of the house?

If you opted to go to the emergency room, you probably had an **electrocardiogram (EKG)**. If you went to your own doctor, however, an EKG might be prescribed, or even performed on the spot if they have the necessary equipment. If you're reading this book and have never had any reason to have an EKG, good for you. You are either one healthy person, fairly young — or you know how to avoid medical situations. Even before heart disease, I had many EKG's. It seems you can't have surgery of any kind without one.

But, to make it very simple: For an EKG, you'll be asked to remove all clothing above your waist. If you're lucky (and many times I have *not* been lucky), you are given at least a paper gown of some sort in an effort to preserve your dignity. You lie down on a table. A number of circular sticky adhesive patches are placed on your ankles, arms, and upper body. (Women: Usually the technician has to move your breast a bit, because one or two of the adhesive patches must be placed strategically under your breasts.) In any case, the testing doesn't take long to perform. If the results are abnormal, however, you may be asked to stay right on that table with those sticky patches on your body until they decide if they wish to redo the test.

An EKG simply measures the electrical activity of the heartbeat. With each beat, an electrical impulse travels through the heart. This impulse causes the heart muscle to squeeze and thus pump blood. The EKG does not hurt. It does not send any electricity into the body. Of course, a slight minor risk could be a skin irritation from those sticky patches, which I seem to get every time.

This simple test can help a doctor determine how long the electrical impulse takes to pass through the heart. The EKG can reveal, among other things:

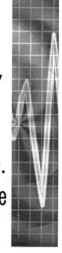

Please be aware that some women have abnormal EKG's, or EKG's that fail to show the presence of early heart disease. This is your time to be your own advocate!

- abnormally fast or irregular heart rhythms;
- abnormally slow heart rhythms;
- abnormal conduction of cardiac impulses (which may suggest underlying cardiac or metabolic disorders);
- evidence of a prior heart attack;
- evidence of an evolving, acute heart attack;
- evidence of an acute impairment in blood flow to the heart during an episode of a threatened heart attack;
- adverse effects on the heart from various heart diseases or systemic diseases, such as high blood pressure and thyroid conditions.

If your test results are normal, then you might have no further need of testing. However, please be aware that some women have abnormal EKG's, or EKG's that fail to show the presence of early heart disease. This is your time to be your own advocate! If you have doubt about the results of your EKG, or if your symptoms continue, have your heart checked out. Again.

Then there is the **Holter monitor**, which is usually prescribed when a patient has heart palpitations (a sensation of fast or irregular heart rhythm). This device works like a portable EKG machine. (I wore one during my visits to cardio rehab.) I highly recommend this test if you feel what you suspect might be symptoms of heart problems — and if those feelings keep happening when you're not at your doctor's office.

The Holter monitor records an EKG continuously for 24-48 hours, then plays back its readings in ultra-fast mode through a computer, allowing the doctor to see the status of the heart at all times during the monitoring period. Amazing, huh? Since the monitor can be worn during your daily activities, it helps the physician correlate symptoms of dizziness, palpitations, or blackouts. This recording over time is much more likely to detect any abnormal heart rhythms than the EKG, which lasts less than a minute. It can also help evaluate the patient's EKG during episodes of chest pain — during which time there may be telltale changes to suggest ischemia (reduced blood supply to the muscle of the left ventricle) — and it may show extra heartbeats, periods of irregular heartbeats, periods of rapid heartbeats called SVT or VT (supraventricular tachycardia or ventricular tachycardia). All of these readings will help your doctor decide if you need further testing.

For me, it was comforting to know that, when I exercised or became agitated, the monitor might be able to give the doctor some signs of what I was experiencing. Request it, if you have any doubt. It's a good test.

Even better, however, is an **Event monitor**. Dr. Johnston prescribed that for me when I became his patient. It was great, too, because the event monitor only has two patches, compared to 12 with the Holter monitor. Event monitors are small, portable devices that can carried in a purse or attached to a belt or shoulder strap like a portable tape or CD player. Event monitors are used to record heart rate and rhythms for longer periods when symptoms are infrequent. The monitors may be carried for several days or even a few weeks. Most monitors are designed to record the heart rate and rhythm only when a button or switch is turned on. For example, when a symptom occurs, the patient can turn on the event recorder, which would then record the heart rate and heart rhythm. The readings can be downloaded over the phone, allowing a cardiologist to determine if there was a problem when the symptoms were occurring.

Now let's say that these initial tests indicate that more testing is required. Maybe, for example, the initial tests showed a high level of LDL (remember that from Chapter 4 — low-density lipoprotein?). As a result, you could be prescribed more **advanced blood tests**, such as the ones I mentioned a few paragraphs earlier — which will show the presence of CRP, Homocysteine, and Lp(a). Elevated levels of CRP (for C-reactive protein), for instance, may provide evidence of arterial inflammation, which has been linked to future cardiovascular events. Homocysteine is an amino acid in the blood. Too much of it is related to a higher risk of coronary heart disease, stroke, or peripheral vascular disease (fatty deposits in the peripheral arteries). Homocysteine may promote atherosclerosis by damaging the inner lining of arteries and promoting blood clots.

If you have checked into the emergency room with the symptoms of a heart attack, then a blood test will show if you have indeed had an attack. How, you ask. Because when you've had a heart attack, cells in the heart die and release enzymes into your bloodstream. Measuring the amount of these markers in the blood can show how much damage was done to your heart. These tests are often repeated at intervals to check for changes. A troponin test, for example, checks the level of this enzyme in the blood. It is considered the most accurate blood test to see if a heart attack has occurred and how much damage was done to the heart. Other diagnostic tests include CK or CK-MB tests and myoglobin tests.

What I learned as a result of these in-depth blood tests was that I had a high level of Lp(a) — often referred to as the "heart attack cholesterol." (Terrific news, huh?) This type of cholesterol is highly genetic and not terribly responsive to diet or exercise. By the way, high Lp(a) readings are *not* an excuse to neglect a healthy regimen of diet or exercise!

Then we have the **noninvasive heart tests**. The first one is usually the **Exercise EKG Test**. It could also be the **Exercise Stress Echocardiography** test (often known as the **stress echo test**) or the **Exercise Stress with Nuclear Imaging**. I lump these tests together for one reason: all three require that you exercise on a treadmill.

The first one I mentioned, the **Exercise and Recording EKG Test**, involves walking on a treadmill set at a higher elevation than you'd normally pick at the gym and recording an exercise EKG. (The technician can raise the elevation, too, as a means of testing your heart's capacity and strength.) This test will detect atherosclerotic narrowing of the heart arteries. You wear the same kinds of patches as if you were having an EKG, but you're exercising instead of lying on a metal table.

Being me, I wore a cute sweatsuit with matching tennis shoes for my first such follow-up test. My very first exposure to this test was in the hospital, where I didn't get to choose my attire. I did learn, however, that you can request hospital-provided pants; maybe it's just me, but I appreciated being able to wear them with my gown. In my own mind, it made my outfit complete and helped me feel more in control of my situation. But let me save you some time. You'll be asked to change into a gown (open at the back, of course); all that would be seen of your cute sweatsuit, I discovered, is about two inches of the legs.

False positives (that is, results that indicate falsely the presence of coronary artery disease) are more common in people who before the test would have been considered to have only a very small chance of having this disease, who are taking certain medications, and who have pre-existing abnormal EKG's. Let me tell you: I can do 30-45 minutes at the gym on a treadmill, but 10 minutes on the treadmill test makes me feel like a perspiring, overweight old woman. Maybe it's a combination of the level of intensity, the incline, and the doctor and nurse standing beside you in case you keel over, but don't feel bad if you have a hard time with this test.

Most important, women seem more likely to register a false positive on this test. False negative tests also occur. Remember that my first test was an exercise stress test in the hospital, and it had only a "slight finding."

> I can do 30-45 minutes at the gym on a treadmill, but 10 minutes on the treadmill test makes me feel like a perspiring, overweight old woman.

The next type of test — the **exercise stress test with echo** — allows the physician to see how the patient's heart is functioning while the patient is engaging in physical exertion. I recommend that women request this test first, if possible. Having the doctor see your heart while you're panting on the treadmill seems to me to be the best option. This test can be useful to determine:

- the extent of a coronary artery blockage;
- the prognosis of patients who have suffered a heart attack;
- the effectiveness of cardiac procedures done to improve circulation in coronary arteries; and
- the cause(s) of chest pain.

Another type of stress test calls for the physician to inject a radioisotope such thallium or cardiolyte into your vein before you walk on the treadmill. (Do not allow this test to be performed if you think you might be pregnant.) This test is particularly useful in patients who have poor echo images, certain types of EKG abnormalities, or severe underlying heart muscle disease.

Here's how the **nuclear stress test** works: When the patient reaches his or her near maximum level of exercise, a small amount of a radioactive substance is injected into the bloodstream. The isotope mixes with the blood in the bloodstream and enters the heart muscle cells. If a part of the heart muscle isn't receiving a normal blood supply, less than a normal amount of the isotope will be found in those cells.

A second picture of the heart, taken after the injection of another dose of the isotope, will be made either before or after the exercise portion of this test when the heart has been at rest.

After exercising, the patient lies down on a special table under a camera that can take pictures of the irradiated blood flowing into the heart muscle. The pictures, made shortly after the exercise test, show blood flow to the heart during exercise. It is an effective way of finding out what's going on inside your heart muscle. If, for example, the test shows that blood flow is normal during rest but not during exercise, then the heart isn't getting enough blood while under stress. If the test is abnormal during both exercise and rest, then there's limited blood flow to that part of the heart at all times, and you may have suffered a heart attack in the past.

A stress test may *not* be recommended for certain patients with known heart disease or other conditions. If you are a patient who may not be able to exercise using the treadmill, you'll still be able to take the test. A drug or pharmacologic agent can be administered to simulate the rapid heartbeat achieved during exercise or alternately to increase blood flow to the heart.

Still another type of test — **Electron Beam Computerized Tomographic (often referred to as EBCT) Imaging** of the coronary artery — is used to detect calcium deposits found in atherosclerotic plaque in the coronary arteries. In the interest of full disclosure, I personally have not had this test; it only became available after I had already been diagnosed with heart disease. There's no reason, in my opinion, to have this test if you've already been diagnosed with coronary artery disease, as I had been.

Amazingly enough, these tests are now offered at all sorts of locations, even at a big mall in our area! If you can afford it, go for it. It's a very simple, non-invasive procedure. State-of-the-art computerized tomography (CT) is the *most* effective way to detect coronary calcification from atherosclerosis, before symptoms develop. I'll repeat that: *before* symptoms develop. More coronary calcium means more coronary atherosclerosis, suggesting a greater likelihood of significant narrowing somewhere in the coronary system and a higher risk of future cardiovascular problems. Your doctor can use the calcium-score to evaluate the risk of future coronary events. Therefore, it's important to realize that certain forms of coronary disease ("soft plaque" atherosclerosis, for example) can escape detection during this CT scan. So you need to know that the CT test may not be able to predict your degree of risk of a life-threatening event such as a heart attack. Nonetheless, don't pass it up if you can afford it.

The 64-Slice CT Scan (MRI Coronary Angiography and CT Coronary Angiography) is the hot new test that you might have seen on "Oprah," as I did. When I saw this testing device featured on such a high-profile TV show, I assumed (mistakenly) that it wasn't available to the general public. I figured that my only option for the most detailed testing would be the traditional "gold standard" test: the **angiography**. However, I've learned that many insurance companies cover this test. Mine did.

During my bout with hyperthyroidism, it was *recommended* that I have the 64-Slice CT Scan rather than the invasive angiogram. It was a spectacular option for me! In reading about this test, I learned that this machine is the most sensitive, accurate CT technology available in the world today — four times more sensitive than the previous generation of devices. If you are at risk for heart disease, stroke, or aortic aneurysm, then having a 64-slice scan can be the answer. This test has the power to reveal problems that can be missed in routine physicals and the early stages of diagnosis.

The 64-slice CT allows for the precise identification of both calcified and non-calcified plaques, and for the early initiation of treatment to prevent heart attacks and sudden cardiac death. Doctors can identify potentially life-threatening coronary artery disease at its earliest stage, without discomfort to the patient because the procedure is noninvasive. This scan also allows patients to find out the cause of unusual symptoms, to check out risk factors due to heredity, or to reassure themselves that they really are healthy.

The examination itself is non-invasive and nearly painless. A small intravenous (IV) catheter will be inserted into a vein in your arm. The so-called "contrast agent" will be injected into this catheter, allowing the doctor to see the images transmitted by the scanner.

Because the best images of the coronary artery are obtained with a heart rate or pulse of 55-70 beats per minute, you may be given a beta blocker about two hours prior to the exam. The goal is for the heart to be as still as possible during the scan, which results in clearer pictures. While waiting for my beta blocker to take effect, I started talking up a storm to the technician about my medical history, and about this book. Both the cardiologist and the technician listened to me in amazement — but I was allowed to sit next to the cardiologist while he viewed my arteries. Admittedly, I could barely tell you what I saw, or what it meant, but my point is that it doesn't hurt to ask to be given a ringside seat.

Your doctor may discuss some of the preliminary findings with you immediately following the exam; however, the results of your scan must be processed by an experienced physician trained to read CT coronary angiography. It usually takes one hour or less from the time you arrive at the imaging center until the exam is completed.

A few details about the test itself: First of all, unlike an MRI scanner, which can be a very claustrophobic experience, the CT scan is a doughnut-shaped structure that does not have this effect. Trust me — I've had both, unfortunately. You lie on what looks a big bed, which slides inside a circular tube. But (and this is a big "but" for me and lots of others who share my claustrophobia) you are not enclosed. The machine itself does the moving, and it really doesn't take long. You do have to change into a gown, but it covered me up well, and my clothes were tucked away in a locker.

During the scan, you are asked to hold your breath for about 10 seconds and to avoid moving. By the way, it's normal to feel a warm sensation for a few seconds when the contrast agent (I just thought of it as plain old dye) is injected. Following your examination, you'll be able to change back into your regular clothes. Oprah would have been proud that her show informed me about this test and that, because of the results of this test, I did not need to have another invasive angiography — which would have been my fourth one.

Angiography is another type of test, but an invasive one. Angiography or arteriography (also called cardiac catheterization) is a medical imaging technique that allows the doctor to get an inside view of your arteries and the chambers of your heart. The image produced by this procedure is called an angiogram.

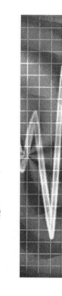

Oprah would have been proud that her show informed me about this test and that, because of the results of this test, I did not need to have another invasive angiography—which would have been my fourth one.

Here's how it works: First they apply a local anesthetic to numb a specific area — usually your right inner groin. Then they make a very small incision there and insert a long thin tube into your femoral artery (one of the largest arteries, it leads directly to your heart). The doctor guides the slender tube all the way to your aorta (the main artery of your body) and into the beginning of your coronary arteries, where a contrast agent is injected.

The purpose of this incredible procedure, of course, is to allow the doctor to see inside your heart and the surrounding blood vessels. If there are blockages that are causing your symptoms, the doctor will be able to see them on a monitor sitting right beside you.

The procedure itself takes an hour or more, but the preparation and recovery time may add several hours. After the procedure, you're required to lie flat for a period of time, and you may receive medication (if you have a PPO) to reduce any discomfort. (Just kidding on the PPO part!) Once you get home, you're not supposed to overexert for a day or two, and to gradually increase your activities until you reach your normal activity level.

In the not-too-distant past, the preferred treatment for blockages due to coronary artery disease (CAD) was a procedure known as **balloon angioplasty**. (I hope I've made it clear that CAD occurs when blood flow to the heart is restricted due to hardened arteries that have become clogged with plaque deposits.)

The goal of balloon angioplasty is to push the fatty plaque back against the artery wall to make more room for blood to flow through the artery. And improved blood flow may reduce the risk of heart attack and sudden cardiac death. Balloon angioplasty was also used as treatment for a heart attack in some emergency facilities. The way this procedure worked was much the same as the angiography I just described. The major difference is that a smaller catheter with a balloon attached is inserted through the diagnostic catheter into the coronary artery. When the balloon-tipped catheter reaches the site of the blockage, the balloon is rapidly inflated, pushing any plaque back against the arterial wall. The catheter is then removed.

These days, though, in most cases the doctor will implant a stent in that spot to hold the artery open. The stent — a little tube made of wire mesh — is fitted over the balloon. When the balloon is inflated, the stent expands and locks in place, forming a kind of scaffold that keeps the artery open. A newer type of stent called a drug-eluting stent gradually releases a drug that helps to keep the artery from closing again.

Other standard treatments for CAD include medication and bypass surgery, which involves constructing little detours around blocked coronary arteries using healthy blood vessels from elsewhere in the body. By the way, bypass surgery is now performed so often in the United States (nearly 500,000 times in 2003, according to the latest data available from the American Heart Association) that the patient may only need to stay in the hospital four to five days afterward.

I'm almost done with my guided tour, but I need to inform you of two other tests — both intended to rule out carotid artery disease. Looking back on what I went through, I certainly understand the need for these tests, though I did not understand at the time. The first was an **MRI of my brain**, which I was told was ordered to check for the presence of transient ischemic attacks, or TIA's, which are actually little strokes that resolve within 24 hours. Not good things to experience, eh? But no one told me why they were doing this test until after the results. Fortunately, my brain MRI showed no presence of brain damage. (Yes, that sounds funny, especially if you know me.)

The other test was the **Doppler ultrasound**, which uses sound waves to check blood flow and measure the thickness of your carotid arteries. This test was quite simple. I laid on a table while what seemed like a microphone went up and down the sides of my neck. This is a great test to see if you are at risk of having a stroke.

The reason I feel it necessary to mention this last part is that strokes are the *number-three killer* in the United States, and a leading cause of disability among older Americans. Also, if you have carotid artery disease, you may also have coronary artery disease. Here are the risk factors for carotid artery disease (note that they are identical to those for coronary artery disease):

- High levels of low-density lipoprotein cholesterol (bad cholesterol) and tri-glycerides in the blood.
- Low levels of HDL (especially in women)
- High blood pressure
- Diabetes
- Smoking
- Family history of premature coronary artery disease
- Obesity
- Lack of exercise

That news should make you go right back to Chapter 4 and do everything in your power to be healthy.

Because my treating cardiologist was stunned to learn that I did indeed have heart disease, he made sure to also test for carotid artery disease. Fortunately, my tests showed no TIA's or blockage. But my larger point in telling you about these tests is to emphasize that we owe it to ourselves to ask questions. Don't have a test performed on you without knowing what it's for.

And with that, my friends, we have completed our stroll down the yellow brick road of diagnostic testing. As I said at the beginning of this chapter, there are only so many tests that can possibly be prescribed for you, and I've had all of them. Knowledge is most certainly power. Somehow it seems right to me to give my mom the last word in this very serious chapter. She's fond of saying, "If you live long enough, you will live long." I think she means that our technology, medications, and treatments keep getting better, so we're lucky to be living in these days of high-tech medicine.

But now I find that I can't leave the last word for anyone else — even my mother! Learn! Ask questions! Inform yourselves. It's your body! Your brain. Your heart.

Chapter 6

My Third Chance at Life

T his won't take me long. If you don't see me clearly by now, then I haven't done my job well enough. Here's the most important thing you need to know about me, Lois Trader: *This is my* third chance *at life*. First came liver disease. Then along came heart disease and altered the whole course of my daily existence. I used to say, smugly, "Only one major sickness per person, per lifetime!" But as the old song said, "It ain't necessarily so."

Because this is my third chance at life, I'm triply grateful for every little blessing that comes my way. And there are so very many blessings. Back to those in a bit, and to why I titled this chapter as I did.

If that fact about me is important for you to understand, here comes the most important single sentence in this little book: Heart disease is the number-one killer of American women. Number one. Numero uno. I know, I know: I've said that already. My excuse for saying it again is that sometimes repetition is called for when a lesson is overwhelmingly important, as this lesson is.

Here are a few vitally important facts for you to take to heart. (Pardon the bad heart humor; it's also part of who I am. Groan.) If you have a heart, heart disease could be a problem for you.

- One in two women in the United States dies of heart disease or stroke; one in 30 dies of breast cancer.
- Thirty-eight percent of women will die within one year after having a heart attack.
- Within six years of having a heart attack, about 46% of women become disabled with heart failure. Two-thirds of those women who suffer a heart attack fail to make a full recovery.
- Coronary heart disease is the number-one killer of American women, but it's also the leading cause of premature, permanent disability in the U.S. labor force, accounting for 19% of disability allowance by the Social Security Administration.

Why are these things true? I believe wholeheartedly that we women don't take ourselves seriously enough. By the time we have been diagnosed with heart disease, our hearts are already deeply compromised.

Women who go to the emergency room with chest pain and are told that it is not caused by a heart attack or angina might want to get a second opinion. Such pains are often ascribed to something else (as was the case with me), but we cannot be content to wait helplessly for the medical community to figure out what's troubling us. We have to be our own advocates and use all the information that is available.

The good news is that heart disease is a problem you can do something about. You have tremendous power to prevent it—and you can start today.

We have to be aware of new symptoms — for instance, unusual fatigue, shortness of breath, and anxiety. I had all those symptoms for over a month, and I see now that they were different, and more severe, than simply being tired or anxious about being late for work. We have to ask about our cholesterol levels and our risk for heart attack and stroke and find out if we need to be on medication.

And then there are all the women who have heart disease and don't want to talk about it. For some reason, heart disease tends to be linked with being old. Trust me, I know. Whenever I wear my "Survivor" T-shirt, I'm always asked if it's because of the TV show. When I respond that I wear the shirt because I have heart disease, the conversation stops cold. Oh, sometimes I'm complimented that I don't look old!

Even after reading this book, you may still be thinking, "This isn't about me. I don't have heart disease." But you may have habits or conditions that can lead to heart disease, such as excess weight, smoking, and not enough physical activity. You may already know these and other risk factors, and you may even know your own risk factors. What you may not know is that if you have even one risk factor, you are much more likely to develop heart disease, with its many serious consequences. A damaged heart can damage your life, interfering with enjoyable activities and even your ability to do simple things, such as taking a walk or climbing steps.

The good news is that heart disease is a problem you can do something about. You have tremendous power to prevent it — and you can start today. By learning about your own personal risk factors and by making healthful changes in your diet, physical activity, and other daily habits, you can greatly reduce your risk of developing heart-related problems. Even if you already have heart disease, you can take steps to lessen its severity.

I have talked to countless hundreds and thousands of women at my seminars. When introduced, I do not allow my introducer to announce me as a woman with heart disease. I start out to overtake the room with my enthusiasm and strength. I share facts about women's heart disease — the same facts I've shared with you. I make eye contact with everyone, including those who are trying hard to look uninterested. Then I carefully tell them about the atypical symptoms I felt and about my terrible experiences in the emergency room during my initial visit.

Once I have their full attention, I know they will listen to how heart disease can affect their own lives.

And what do I tell them? Why, that heart disease is the number-one killer of American women, of course! No, I am never fearful that my seminars will be ill-attended or that I will have trouble getting the attention of younger women. Women, because they are women, relate to another woman, no matter what the age difference, when she talks about the heart by showing her own heart. When it comes to this vitally important topic, there are no meaningful differences that can be caused by age, size, ethnicity, or social or marital status. All women are equal — and equally in danger — when it comes to this topic.

Each time I share my story, women approach me afterwards and open their hearts. They share about relatives with heart disease. Some divulge secretly, as if ashamed, that they have heart disease themselves. Women tell, knowing their own family history, that they live in fear. They tell me that they appreciate the encouragement I give them to stand strong and go back to their doctors armed with information from one who has been there.

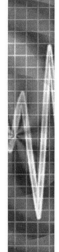

Women have the gift of intuition. Use it. We know our own bodies, and we know—somewhere inside us—when something isn't right. We need to take the time to listen and take care of ourselves.

I tell women, again and again: Trust yourselves. Listen to what your body is trying to tell you. Know the facts.

One time I found myself playing the role of the "heart attack survivor guest" on a national TV show. Beside me sat a so-called expert on heart disease (I'll name no names here). After hearing a five-minute version of my experience in the emergency room, the host asked, "When do we know it's the 11th hour, time to deal with our symptoms?" The expert answered (before I could), "If you are under 50 years old, you are protected from heart disease." As I tried to maintain my composure in the face of such glaring misinformation, he added that women of child-bearing age need not worry about heart disease. (Maybe, I thought, he's a colleague of the doctor I saw in the emergency room — the one who prescribed antacids and sent me home.)

Wow, I ranted to myself, my 20-year-old daughter can stop taking her statin! (Statins are a class of drugs used to lower blood cholesterol. They work in your liver to block a substance needed to make cholesterol. They may also help your body re-absorb cholesterol that has accumulated in plaques on your artery walls.) And now she doesn't need to worry that her bad cholesterol numbers are off the chart! Plus I can save over $600 a year on her medications! Hooey.

After the TV show had been taped, and after the so-called expert had departed, I shared with the producers and the host the same information that I have shared with you. In other words, the medical expert was dead wrong. On my way to the airport I answered my cell phone and was delighted that the producers asked me to come back and tape another show. No "experts" this time — just me. Job well done.

Hear me, please. It *does* matter if your father, uncle, or grandmother had heart disease. Ignorance is *not* bliss; it can be fatal. From my own personal experience, nine out of 10 of the women I speak to do not know (or have not accepted) that heart disease is a very real danger in their lives.

Women have the gift of intuition. Use it. We know our own bodies, and we know — somewhere inside us — when something isn't right. We need to take the time to listen and take care of ourselves. One last time, the common heart disease symptoms include shortness of breath, fatigue, chest or back discomfort or pain that can spread to the arms, neck, back, or jaw. Many of these symptoms occur during periods of physical activity or stress. You should tell your health-care provider about any worri-some or annoying symptoms that you experience, *especially* those that are new. Re-member, though, that many women with heart disease experience no symptoms at all, which is why regular checkups are so important. So listen to your body. *You* must do it. No one can do it for you.

Finally, since the symptoms of heart attack can be different in women than in men, women may not recognize their symptoms and may delay getting to the hospital for treatment. Once they get to the hospital, they are often not given prompt or appro-priate treatments for a heart attack. Therefore, you *must* be your own advocate. Learn from my experience. Take steps today to change your life.

Back to the importance of blessings. Though I've joked about taking care of my-self, I really have made many changes to my lifestyle. Major changes, in fact. None of these changes have killed me (whew!), but without these changes I would likely be killing myself. Each day challenges me to incorporate these changes, and to be good to my body. Yes, life is precious, and when you hear someone say, "Life goes so quickly," please take it to heart. I do. Literally.

In this, my third chance at life, I notice everything. I'm acutely aware of how I reacted before to, say, a dirty kitchen — how easily I would allow this and countless other minor annoyances to get the best of me. Now I rarely find anything upsetting enough to warrant an outburst of anger; when I do, I realize that I'm wasting precious moments of life. The Serenity Prayer has become very real to me:

> God grant me the serenity to accept the things I cannot change,
> The courage to change the things I can,
> And the wisdom to know the difference.

Serenity had not been a part of my life. I had to look it up in the dictionary! Serenity: calmness, peacefulness, composure, coolness (my favorite). I want to be cool! I can't change the fact that I have heart disease. I can't change other people. But I *can* change me.

In this third life of mine, I long to spend more time with my mom and her husband. Mothers and daughters have rare relationships. We are so much to each other — more than a friend could ever be. I understand so much more now about how helpless my mom felt about my illnesses and not being able to fix them for me. I am learning to deal with seeing her new age-related challenges, and I want to be a strong and healthy daughter for her and her husband (she remarried many years ago, to a wonderful man), just as they have always been there for me and my children.

My mother is my inspiration. A few months after my heart attack, she accompanied me to the cardiologist. My mom told him that she was extremely healthy; she asked if it would help me if she gave me her arteries or veins. Think about what I just wrote. She was offering her life for mine. How much more blessed could I be?

I'm proud of my three daughters and the lives they're creating for themselves. Every time Bethany's strong healthy 2-year-old calls me "Ga Ga," it's worth every minute it takes me to swallow my pills, to drive to the gym, to say no to that piece of cake I don't need. Learning, in my newfound serenity (at least most of the time!) to allow Cortney and her husband to create their own life as a couple, and to be thankful that I'm here to appreciate them. Seeing Michal graduate from college, and enjoying her friendship as she grows into a young woman.

I'm so proud of all three of my girls, but I'm learning not to define myself by them, and not to define myself by my heart disease. Instead, I define myself as one who is becoming a better human being, a more caring and accepting person. Which brings me to accepting my husband Tim's unconditional love through sickness and health. I rejoice in the fact that we made choices along the way to stay partners, when we could have chosen not to do so. My heart overflows with warmth and happiness. I'm excited that I get to grow old with husband, my buddy, my friend.

I take the time to sit outside. My husband says the birds are my birds. I drop bird-seed everywhere so they will enjoy the backyard with us. Enjoying my girlfriends and taking the time to nurture those relationships. Drinking a glass of wine to end my day, saying a little prayer, "Help me learn to relax, give me peace with my past, and contentment with where and who I am today." I love daydreaming, planning my future to include barbecues with my grandchildren, laughing with my daughters and their own families.

Oh, and yes, accepting a few extra pounds and some new wrinkles, and not minding it when someone tells me I look good for my age. Yes, my age. I'm here — and I'm so terribly thankful to be here.

The phone rings. It's the cardiologist's office confirming my appointment for tomorrow. And so, my new friends, be aware of the battle we have with our hearts. Take care. Trust your intuition. Make the time to sit down with your doctor, and make the time to sit down with yourself. Throw a couple of extra dishes of vegetables on the table. Most of all, love yourself. You'll do your heart a lot of good.

With that, I must put on my walking shoes, grab an apple, and say good-bye.

Epilogue 1

Danielle!

Throughout this book there has been a missing piece to my story: my dear brother Richard's little girl Danielle. In Chapter 3 I told you that Richard committed suicide when I was 20; he was 26 years old. Living was harder for him than dying. Why, we never knew for certain.

You know, too, that Richard was married at the time, and his baby Danielle was only a year old. In the months following Richard's death, we would pick up Danielle on the weekends. I'd watch my parents sit for hours and play with her. I recall so clearly Danielle bouncing on my bed while my dad laid on his side, watching and watching his only grandchild.

But one Saturday, when my parents went to pick her up, Danielle and her mother were gone. Much later we found out that Richard's widow had used his death-benefit payment to buy a car and take a long trip. We were never able to locate them. It was another horrible blow to all of us — but especially to my parents.

Years passed, and my father died in a Hong Kong hotel room, as I told you, and again we tried to locate Danielle. Again, no luck.

Fast forward to February 2005. All these years later, seeing my mom still grieving for Richard, I promised myself that I would find Danielle, in the hope that she would want to be part of our family. For years I had considered using a search company, but had not felt the time was right. Now, however, I hired a company to find her, even though I had very little information to assist them in the search. At the end of one of the busiest weeks of my life, speaking to women about heart disease, I picked up the mail and plopped down on the couch, exhausted.

There it was: a letter from the company I had contacted a month earlier, stating confidently that my niece, Danielle (Stewart) Woods, lived just an hour away! They even gave me her address and phone number. I stared at the letter, astounded. What would she look like? Would she be happy to hear from me? Or a terribly unhappy person who wouldn't want to talk to me?

Those thoughts lasted only seconds. I don't think I stopped to breathe; I just dialed the phone number. The sweetest-sounding young girl answered the phone, and I began talking quickly, before I could think.

"Hi, Danielle, I don't know if you knew you had a dad named Richard Stewart, but

I'm his sister Lois. I love you, I have always loved you, my girls love you, we have always wanted to find you. . . ."

She broke in: "Is your mom alive?" she asked.

"Yes, your grandmother is alive and she wants to know you, see you, and be a part of your life. She always has. We've never been able to find you."

Danielle told me she is married, with a baby girl, and that she wanted to get to know all of us. She also said that she had been told about her father when she was 8 years old. We arranged for her to come to my house the following weekend. As we spoke, I could feel the years of separation begin to melt away.

Then I told her urgently, "Danielle, I need you to understand about the heart disease that runs in our family." She stunned me by replying that she had already suffered a heart attack two years before, when she was 28. Since the heart attack, Danielle has had to deal with pericarditis, which is a swelling and irritation of the pericardium, the thin sac-like membrane surrounding the heart.

The most common symptom of pericarditis is sharp, stabbing pain behind the breastbone or in the left side of the chest. A minority of people with this condition describe their chest pain as dull, achy, or pressure-like instead, and of varying intensity. The sharp pain may travel into your left shoulder and neck, and often intensifies when you lie down or inhale deeply. Sitting up and leaning forward can often ease the pain. At times, it may be difficult to distinguish pericardial pain from the pain of a heart attack.

And get this: Four days later, Danielle wrote me this e-mail: "I just went to my cardiologist today and got a clean bill of health. My heart attack could probably have been prevented if my doctor at the time wasn't such a boob — one of those dismissive 'you're too young for this to be a heart attack' types. The funny thing is that I always said it felt like there was an elephant stepping on my chest. That doctor would say, 'Nurse, she's having an asthma attack.'"

Can you believe what Danielle wrote: "I always said it felt like there was an elephant stepping on my chest." Yep, she's my niece.

I hung up from talking to Danielle and called my mom. I had dreamed of this moment.

"Mom, are you sitting down?" I began. "Really, are you sitting down? Mom, I found Danielle, and she asked first thing if you were alive. She wants to see us, and she's coming over next weekend. She's married, with a baby girl, Mom. You have another great-grandchild."

Silence on the other end of the line, and then my mother said, "I must be there when she comes for the first time." Yes, of course. After all, I had done this for her.

That next weekend, a beautiful, tiny, 30-year-old woman walked through our front door — small, with lots of freckles like my oldest daughter. She looked just like my girls! There was Richard's dear face, his nose, our family's deep brown eyes, the same skin and eye coloring as my own daughters. And such a loving smile. . .

Together, with my girls at our side, we walked into the living room, where my mom sat waiting. It was like a scene from a movie — surreal, unbelievable, beautiful. There she was — Danielle, our lost baby we hadn't seen since she was almost 2 years old — hugging my mom and her kind husband, the only grandfather my girls have ever known. I felt so strongly that we had all become deeply joined, finally, with Richard.

And I felt my father there beside us.

I see this last piece of the puzzle — this gift of returning Danielle to my mother — as a kind of emblem of my mission: to help heal women's hearts, inside and out. If you touch one life, you touch a million. I believe that with all my own wounded and healing heart, and I witnessed it that day.

And, really, it's eerie, isn't it? That my life's work is to share with women about heart disease, and my long-lost niece comes back into our lives, with her own heart challenges. It all fits together, doesn't it?

Last of all, here's something for you to ponder, my new friends. Later on the same day that I first called Danielle, my mother reminded me that it was Richard's birthday, February 4, which is also the anniversary of his death. For me to find Danielle and contact her on her father's birthday was almost too much to handle. Almost. But having Richard's baby girl back in our lives makes anything bearable, don't you think?

Epilogue 2

My Dream

If you know someone with heart disease, it's easy to think something that terrible will certainly never happen to you. Take me, for example: I absolutely know I have heart disease (and now so do you), but almost two years after the discovery of my own heart disease, I still needed to make a separate appointment with my cardiologist just to make sure! I thought that maybe if I asked him in a different way, I'd get a different answer.

The whole process that I've been through — learning about women's heart disease, learning about my own heart disease, and slowly coming to accept that I'll have heart disease for the rest of my life — is terribly hard to put into daily perspective. Somehow I find it much easier to write about, and to speak about, than to actually grasp completely for myself.

I keep wondering what happened. In a moment, an actual heartbeat in time, everything in my life was forever changed. I feel as if I became a new person. But that new person whose story you've been reading has found an unexpected depth of healing in helping others. Speaking to groups of women has helped me more than I could possibly have imagined. I'm always thanked by women for coming to speak with them, but I'm the one who is appreciative.

Often I receive calls after a seminar from someone who heard me speak, then went immediately and saw her doctor. One woman told me that what I shared about my symptoms prompted her to convince her mother to see a doctor. Within a week of my seminar, her mom was having a procedure for blocked arteries. They are forever grateful, as I am honored to have been able to help them.

I have named my seminars "Healing the Whole Heart," and I prepare for them with quiet time. Quiet time is something I have to strive to achieve. Sometimes that quiet time becomes very like a reverie, a dream. And the dream is always the same. Dream along with me. . .

Picture a boxing match. We're all in a big stadium. I'm in one corner, holding this book. In the other corner is my opponent, Women's Heart Disease.

My robe and shorts are bright red — the color chosen by the American Heart Association to represent women's heart disease. My shorts have the word *Surviving* embroidered on the waistband. In my corner are closest friends and family — and my trainer/editor and a cut man because I fall a lot, sometimes from exhaustion, occasionally due to finances. Sometimes I confess that I have so much self-doubt that my legs buckle under me from weakness. I rely strongly on each of my supporters; they know that this match is being fought for the millions of women who will be tuning in to watch.

Turning around, I see the stands are filled with women, cheering women — about 500,000 of them. Probably 25% of the rows are filled with women who died from Sudden Cardiac Arrest (SCA). These women cry out to encourage me. They seem to be the saddest group — maybe because they didn't get a chance to tell their loved ones good-bye. They left grocery lists on the fridge, children at soccer practice, and nothing thawed for dinner. They left business proposals unsigned and bills unpaid. When they saw their death certificates that read "cause of death SCA," sadness and guilt overwhelmed them.

When I falter, I cry out. But I get up again. I always get up again.
Because the work ahead of me — the women's lives waiting
to be saved — is too important to quit.

"Keep telling your story wherever you go," they cry out to me in my dream. "Please continue writing and sharing with women. Someone has to tell our daughters, sisters, and girlfriends." Another group, sobbing tears of regret, calls to me: "We should have listened to our intuition. It really wasn't sudden. We suspected for months that something was wrong. We had been out of breath when we walked the stairs, knew we needed to slow down, needed to make an appointment with our doctor."

All these women — row upon row, stretching up and back farther than I can see — look so different. So many races and colors sitting together! Like a rainbow, the rows stretch back, filled with beautiful shades of skin tones. These women are chanting: "Tell them, Lois! Tell them about all the risks, including diabetes. Go over all the risk factors. Warn them!"

Many of these women died because of complications from diabetes. When first diagnosed with diabetes, they didn't worry that it could affect their heart too. They talk quickly, almost drowning one another out, but I hear the message: "If we had known the risks, we would have been more careful with our diets, taken our medication for high blood pressure, checked our cholesterol, and made the time to exercise."

Another cheering section is yelling: "We love it when you make us laugh! Laughter is healing." And another group in the huge arena shouts: "We love it when you talk about fiber and how we don't have to conquer every change overnight. But if we had just incorporated a little change in our lives daily, maybe. . ." Their voices drift into silence.

Then quietly, almost in a whisper, I hear a younger woman's voice say, "I thought I was protected during my child-bearing years, so I figured I'd stop smoking when I turned 40." Somehow the small voice sounds familiar, and silently I pray it's not one of my daughters. Then I see the girl, and she's the same age as my oldest daughter. This lovely young woman clears her throat and tells me, "I miss my children so much. My little girl is only 5, and my baby boy just turned 3. Please tell everyone that heart disease doesn't care what we wear, or what age we are. Tell them now."

I close my eyes and the cries die away. *Half a million women*, I think to myself. *Half a million deaths each year that might have been prevented.* And I gain renewed strength from knowing that my story can make it possible for wives to remain with their husbands, mothers with their young children, and their children's children.

Then I begin to speak again. And when I falter, I cry out. But I get up again. I always get up again. Because the work ahead of me — the women's lives waiting to be saved — is too important to quit.

I am Lois Trader, a woman with heart disease.

Afterword

Women and Heart Disease: The Hidden Epidemic

by Dr. Warren D. Johnston

If you are a woman, it would not be surprising if you thought that cancer — specifically, breast cancer — is the biggest threat to your future health. It also would not be surprising if you felt that heart disease is largely a man's disease. **Wrong and Wrong!** The truth of the matter is that your biggest health risk is indeed heart disease. Furthermore, heart disease is more of a risk for women than for men. In the paragraphs that follow, I'll try to bring you up to speed with the epidemic of heart disease in women, and how, until fairly recently, it has been hidden from the perception of most American women.

First, let's discuss what exactly cardiovascular disease is. Cardiovascular disease refers to the disease process called atherosclerosis, which is the infiltration of major arteries in the body with fat, cholesterol, scar and other tissue, which over a period of time can slowly begin to block blood flow through the channel of the artery. This disease can affect the arterial supply of the heart (the coronary arteries), as well as the arteries that supply the brain (the carotid arteries), and can also affect the arteries that supply the legs, causing peripheral vascular disease.

Here I will primarily discuss coronary artery disease — that is, the disease process which blocks off the arteries that supply the heart muscle with blood. There are three major manifestations of coronary artery disease. The first is angina, which is chest pain or discomfort caused by the blocked artery. The second is myocardial infarction, sometimes referred to as a heart attack, where a coronary artery is nearly or completely blocked off, causing the heart muscle supplied by that artery to, in fact, die. Lastly, coronary artery disease can present as sudden death.

Interestingly, if one examines how people present with coronary artery disease for the very first time, it has been shown that for 25% of individuals, they experience sudden death. Fifty percent of individuals will experience a heart attack (myocardial infarction) with irreversible heart damage. Only 25% of people display the symptoms of angina (that is, chest discomfort), warning them of the presence of this lethal disease. This is a disease process which begins early in life, often in the first decade, and can proceed inexorably through life leading to sudden death, as mentioned above, or myocardial infarction unless it is discovered early and treated appropriately.

Cardiovascular disease affects a large percentage of our population. One in every five people in the United States has some form of cardiovascular disease. Cardiovascular disease claims nearly one million lives every year and accounts for 40% of all deaths in the U.S. Some 1.1 million people suffer heart attacks every year. Cardiovascular disease accounts for 15% to 32% of all of our nation's health-care costs.

Until recently, cardiovascular disease was considered mainly a man's disease. Nothing could be further from the truth! In fact, cardiovascular disease became the number-one killer of women in 1908. In fact, since 1985, more women have died of cardiovascular disease than men.

What are the facts regarding women and cardiovascular disease? Some 43% of all female deaths in the U.S. occur from cardiovascular disease. One in every five U.S. women has some form of cardiovascular disease. One in seven women between the ages of 45 to 64 has cardiovascular disease. One in three women age 65 or above has cardiovascular disease. In women ages 25 to 44, cardiovascular disease is the third leading cause of death. In the U.S., cardiovascular disease is the most common diagnosis when women are discharged from the hospital.

Other startling facts regarding cardiovascular disease in women are that women are *six times* more likely to die of a heart attack than of breast cancer. Women are twice as likely to die of cardiovascular disease than from all forms of cancer combined. Disturbingly, 38% of women (versus 25% of men) die within the first year of a heart attack. Of further concern, 63% of women who die suddenly of coronary artery disease had no previous symptoms.

Despite these facts, women's perceptions of their health threats are clearly quite different. In fact, in polls of women in the United States, 55% of women felt that their biggest health threat was cancer, with 40% of women thinking they would die of breast cancer. Only 22% of women perceived that heart disease was a threat to them, and only 2% of women felt they could die of a heart attack.

There have been historical misperceptions in the medical profession which have underscored our misunderstanding of the risk of heart disease in women. Many (if not most) physicians felt that heart disease was a man's disease. Indeed, enrollments in clinical trials until recently have included very few women. Thus research on diagnosis and treatment of heart disease has virtually been confined to a male population.

And thus our knowledge of heart disease in women has been rather poor. This has led to both underdiagnosis and undertreatment of women. This less aggressive care has resulted in higher complications and death rates for our women patients.

In discussing cardiovascular disease, it is quite important to understand the risk factors for development of this disease. Risk factors are typically identified as modifiable versus non-modifiable. Modifiable risk factors include hypertension, abnormal cholesterol levels, diabetes, cigarette smoking, obesity, and physical inactivity. Non-modifiable risk factors include family history (i.e., your genetics), age, and gender. Again, in past years when we discussed gender, being a male was identified as being a risk factor, when clearly being a female is an even bigger risk factor.

It will not come as a surprise for most of you reading this article that men and women are different. In fact, if "men are from Mars and women are from Venus," it would make sense that women might well have different risk factors, different presentations of the disease, and potentially different outcomes when they do develop heart disease.

Relative to risk factors, it has been shown that there is a higher prevalence of increased blood cholesterol, of physical inactivity, and of obesity in the female population in the United States compared to men. As another example, diabetes is a more powerful risk factor for cardiovascular disease in women than in men. There is a risk from three to seven times greater of cardiovascular disease in women diabetics versus a risk from two to three times greater in male diabetics. It has also been shown that low levels of good cholesterol (HDL) in women are much more predictive of the development of cardiovascular disease than similarly low levels of HDL in men.

The sad fact is that women are counseled less about risk-factor reduction, as well as nutrition, exercise, and weight control. They are also treated less aggressively to reduce risk factors, such as hypertension, diabetes, and hypercholesterolemia.

Another risk factor that stands out is smoking. Smoking is the single most preventable cause of death in the United States. Here again, women are different. Smoking by women causes 150% more deaths from heart disease than does lung cancer. Women who smoke are two to six times more likely to suffer heart attacks. Ironically, while the prevalence of smoking is decreasing in the U.S., the only group in which it is increasing is among teenage women.

Gender differences certainly apply to how women display the symptoms of heart disease. Women clearly present in a much more atypical fashion than men. Having said that, it is important for all genders to understand the symptoms that you might develop if, in fact, you are experiencing angina or a heart attack for the first time. You may well experience pain, pressure, and squeezing or a stabbing discomfort in your chest. That pain may radiate to the neck, shoulder, back, arm, or jaw. You might undergo a pounding heart rate or a change in heart rhythm. You might notice shortness of breath or difficulty in breathing. A not infrequent symptom is that of heartburn, nausea, vomiting, or abdominal pain. This leads to the expression: "Is this heartburn or a heart attack?" It is not unusual to experience clamminess or to sweat profusely. These symptoms are common to both sexes.

Women, however, can display quite different symptoms. Often, if not frequently, the symptoms are much milder and may not include actual chest pain. Women can present with the sudden onset of weakness, shortness of breath, fatigue, body aches, and an overall feeling of illness. Women can also experience an unusual feeling of mild discomfort in the back, chest, arm, neck, or jaw — again without chest discomfort.

In surveys done in emergency rooms looking at how men and women display cardiovascular disease, it has been found that women are much more likely to experience shortness of breath, nausea, vomiting, fatigue, sweating, or arm or shoulder pain. On the other hand, men are more likely to experience chest discomfort in the substernal or breastbone area.

Because of the misperception that cardiovascular disease is primarily a man's disease, it has been shown that in patients referred for stress-testing who subsequently have a positive test suggesting that they might well have cardiovascular disease, *many more women than men receive no follow-up testing*. In this population of women and men with positive stress tests, women are much more likely to experience cardiac death or a heart attack. Sadly, women have been shown to be less frequently referred for coronary artery bypass grafting or balloon angioplasty. This situation is intolerable.

Happily, there is now a national initiative to rectify this situation. The American Heart Association has begun the "Go Red for Women" campaign with the intention of educating every woman in the United States regarding their risks of developing heart disease. First Lady Laura Bush has adopted heart disease in women as one of her national initiatives. She has started the "Heart Truth Campaign," using the red dress as a symbol of women's vulnerability to heart disease.

I am the Medical Director of the Women's Heart Center at St. Joseph Hospital in Orange, California. We were the first women's heart center in Orange County, California. Working with the American Heart Association and the Heart Truth Campaign, our mission is to educate women about the prevalence of heart disease, and to intervene in a manner appropriate to the differences in a woman's heart.

Women entering the Women's Heart Center are first given a cardiovascular risk questionnaire; their risk of developing heart disease is quantified using a scoring system developed from the Framingham Study. They are then screened for cardiovascular risk factors by obtaining a fasting lipid profile, a fasting blood sugar, a blood pressure measurement, and an assessment of their body weight obtained through a body mass index measurement. Women who are identified as having significant risk factors are counseled on lifestyle modification, including diet, exercise, and weight loss. Women who are found to have high cholesterol, hypertension, or diabetes are treated with appropriate lifestyle modifications and pharmaceutical treatment. Women smokers are counseled regarding cessation of smoking, and are given the opportunity to participate in pharmacotherapy for smoking cessation purposes. Women are also be given appropriate hormonal replacement counseling.

The first "Go Red for Women Day" was in February 2004. The 2005 and 2006 anniversaries of "Go Red for Women Day" resulted in an impressive outpouring of recognition of a woman's risks of cardiovascular disease. I encourage you to wear the "Go Red for Women" pin year round. Please support your American Heart Association in its efforts to enhance the knowledge of the risk of cardiovascular disease in women and in its efforts to raise funds for further research into ending the plague of cardiovascular disease in both men and women in the United States.

Warren D. Johnston, MD, FACC, FACP, is board certified in internal medicine, cardiovascular disease, and geriatric medicine. He is a 15-year partner with the Cardiology Specialists of Orange County specializing in noninvasive and invasive cardiology, the Medical Director of the Women's Heart Center at St. Joseph Hospital, Orange, California, founded in 2003, and Assistant Clinical Professor in Cardiology at the University of California, Irvine Medical School. Dr. Johnston is president of the Orange County Chapter of the American Heart Association. He has participated in many research projects, written numerous articles, and is a frequently requested lecturer.